A Family Guide To Covid

Questions & Answers for Parents, Grandparents and Children

SECOND EDITION

D1456596

William A. Haseltine PhD

Thank you for buying the Family Guide to Covid! This is what we call a *living book*. As our understanding of the disease changes, so will the contents of this book—and as its owner, you now have a permanent pass to every edition to come.

Visit www.accessh.org/covidfamilyguide

Click on Read The Book

And enter the password: AskDrBill

You'll be taken to a special section of our website where you can download the most up to date version.

You can also contribute to future editions of the book by clicking on *Ask Dr. Bill A Question* and asking me anything I didn't cover. Your question might just appear in the next edition, or in the question and answer section of our website.

I look forward to hearing from you!

Sincerely,

Dr. Bill

P.S. I earned the Dr. in my title when I earned my Ph.D. If you have questions about the virus that causes Covid or about the disease itself, I am probably the right person to ask. But if you have specific questions about an illness or a treatment, you should seek advice from a medical doctor instead.

To my children, Mara and Alexander, who triumph now as always over illness.

To my loving wife, Maria Eugenia, and her tireless efforts to care for us all.

To my step-daughters, Karina, Manuela, and Camila, each a model of loving care and responsibility.

To our three grandchildren, Pedro Agustin, Enrique Matias, and Carlos Eduardo, may they live in a peaceful and healthy world.

And to parents and grandparents everywhere, who are helping their children learn and grow through this difficult time.

CONTENTS

PREFACE TO THE SECOND EDITION

The first edition of the Family Guide to Covid was published only a few weeks ago—and yet the world already looks so different. Not a day has passed where we didn't lose someone to this disease. Nor has a day gone by where we didn't learn something new about it.

Below are just a few examples of what's new in the second edition:

A bonus section on summer safety, complete with six brand new illustrations and tips for kids and adults alike (page 161)

Questions and answers for new mothers and mothers-to-be, based on the latest research into connections between Covid and pregnancy (page 92)

Guidance on how to determine risk, especially for those of us living in areas where lockdown has ended but new cases persist (page 31)

Asterisks (*) indicate questions and answers that have been newly updated, while daggers (†) indicate questions and answers newly added. I hope this living book can continue to offer clarity and comfort in the face of the uncertainty we all feel, today and in the months to come.

July 2020

INTRODUCTION

A new disease has spread across our world. Schools have shut down, people around the world have been asked to stay home, businesses have shuttered, and economies are crashing.

The sad state of affairs is not entirely new to me. I remember how polio overshadowed my younger years. Swimming, my favorite relief from the oppressive heat of the Mojave Desert where I was raised, was forbidden. So too were the cool dark theaters where I longed to see the latest Flash Gordon and Hopalong Cassidy films.

With time, I realized that diseases don't just harm individuals, but rather cripple communities and devastate entire countries. I eventually became a scientist, dedicating my life to understanding the diseases that threaten us most and figuring out ways to stop and prevent them.

Today, I find that my children, my grandchildren, many of my friends, and extended family members are coming to me with question after question. Why have our lives changed? Are my children in danger? When will this be over? Will there be a vaccine or a cure and, if so, when? When will our lives return to normal?

I've earned the nickname 'Willapedia' because of the odd bits of knowledge I've collected from reading, traveling, and talking to people who know a lot more than I do. I have studied diseases and modern medicine with a laser-like focus and written many books. I have made profound discoveries about how living systems work and deciphered the secrets of another great plague known as HIV/AIDS. I created companies that have brought drugs to market to treat and prevent cancer, AIDS, diabetes, and lupus. I have developed vaccines and ways to thwart potential bioweapons like anthrax. I have worked to help strengthen health systems around the world. And I have had a great time doing it, working with some of the greatest minds of our time, and with friends from all walks of life and on every continent.

I have dedicated my life to making sure everyone, no matter where they live, no matter what their age, has access to high-quality affordable health care. My friends and colleagues know I am plainspoken, and I don't pull my punches when I see truth.

This book attempts to answer questions about Covid honestly, with equal measures of clarity and compassion. It is written especially for those of you who are faced with the difficult task of not only protecting yourselves, but of protecting your families, your children, your spouses, and your parents.

The first section answers questions your children and grandchildren may ask. Each of the questions in this section are ones that I have been asked by the younger people in my life, some as young as four and five.

The second section provides short answers to many of the difficult questions that adults from ages eighteen to one hundred ask themselves to understand this new reality. Again, these are real questions people have asked. The answers are as concise and straightforward as I could make them. For those who want to know more, I will add a link to what I view as being reliable sources that will allow questioning readers to judge the answers for themselves.

Our understanding of the pandemic, what is it, and where it is going is changing almost daily. The burning questions of today may not be those of tomorrow. Even the answers to the same question may change. That is why this will be an ever-changing manuscript, a book that will be updated as new questions and new answers appear. You can access the most up to date version of the book by visiting www.accessh.org/covidfamilyguide and entering the password "AskDrBill". The printed version of the book will also be updated regularly on Amazon.

In my heart and soul, I am a scientist, one who has devoted his life to discovering new ways to treat and cure disease and to make sure all who walk this earth share the benefits of science and medicine. I am certain that science will show us the way, that in the end science will save us as it has done so many times before, from the likes of smallpox to the bubonic plague, polio and so many other great scourges of the past.

In the meantime, we must fight this disease in our homes, in our communities, and in our hospitals with the tools we have: vigilance, self-isolation, public health measures, and the best care for those who are ill.

Our children and grandchildren will one day look back, as I do, and remember a time when disease stalked the streets and changed their life. I hope some of those children will be inspired to dedicate their lives to science and medicine so that their own children and grandchildren will never have to endure what they did.

June 2020

PART ONE

Questions Kids Ask Us

Let's start with the first and most basic question I'm often asked:

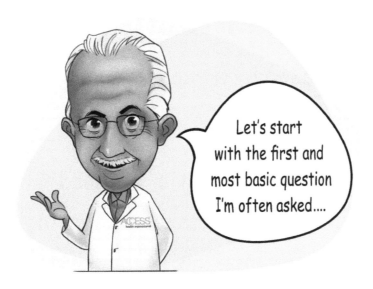

Let's start with the first and most basic question I'm often asked....

Why has my life changed?

There is a new disease going around that is dangerous. Some people who catch it get very sick.

Right now, no vaccine can prevent someone from catching it. And no medicine can cure it.

Our job is to keep you safe. The best way to do that is to keep you at home so you can't catch the disease. Once we think it is safe, you can meet up with your friends again and go back to school.

Why is the disease called Covid?

The disease is caused by a super tiny germ called a *virus*.

Covid is short for *coronavirus.*

This virus has a lot of spikes on its surface that makes it look like a crown. *Corona* means crown in Latin, the old language that scientists use to name lots of things. Corona + virus = coronavirus. And *coronavirus disease* = Covid.

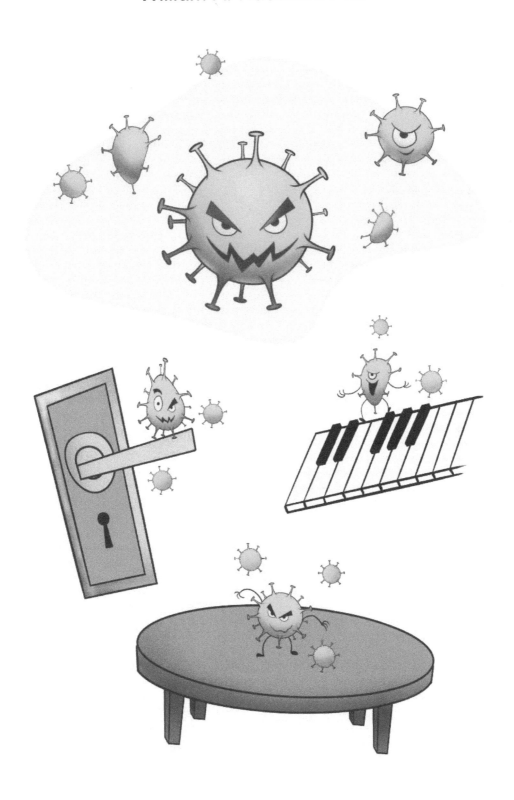

How do people catch the disease?

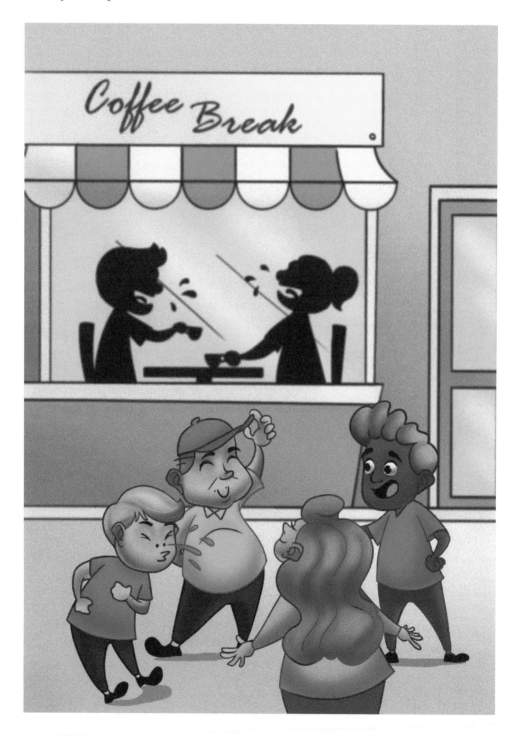

You catch it just like you catch a cold: by being around people who have it.

If someone in your school has a cold, chances are you will get it. It is the same for this disease. When people sneeze, cough, and even talk, they spread germs. If you are near them, those germs can land on you.

Some of the objects around you may have germs on them too, like a doorknob that a sick person touched or a pencil they put in their mouth.

You may also catch it from drinking or swimming in dirty water.

What does this disease do to the body to make us so sick?

When little viruses invade the body, they begin to make lots of copies of themselves so they can take over. This coronavirus is good at getting inside our lungs, especially in older people. When the virus grows deep inside the lungs, it gets harder to breathe. The body can even start to shut down, which is why some people need to be hooked up to special machines that breathe for them.

How small is the virus?

The virus is so tiny that hundreds and hundreds of them could fit on the head of a needle.

Can the virus attack parts of the body other than the lungs?

Yes, it can get in your nose and throat. It can also get in your blood vessels, your heart and your intestines.

How does the body fight the disease?

Your body has a defense system that protects you at all times. Your body has seen most germs before, so when they attack, your defense system can kick them out easily.

Others take a little longer to battle, and a little more power, too. That's why you sometimes get fevers—your defense system is working hard to clear bad germs out of your body.

How do I avoid catching it?

Stay inside as much as possible. It's easier for us to protect ourselves at home than outside, where germs are floating all around us.

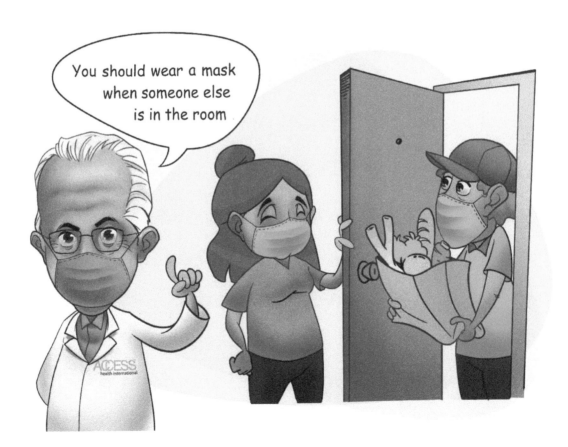

If you do go outside, *stay a safe distance* away from other people. If you see somebody you know on the street, you can smile and wave, but don't get close to them.

Wash your hands—a lot. If germs get on your hands, drowning them in soap and water may be able to kill them.

This is why you should also *avoid touching your face.* Especially your eyes, your nose, and your mouth. Don't pick your nose or suck your thumb! It is easier to wash the virus off your hands than off your face.

How do I wash my hands properly?

Get your hands super wet and super soapy. Then rub your hands together for a whole 20 seconds. You can sing "Happy Birthday" out loud or in your head twice as a way to keep the time. Make sure you rub soap onto the backs of your hands, the palms of your hands, between your fingers, your thumbs, and even underneath your fingernails.

When you're done singing "Happy Birthday", rinse all the soap off. Shake, shake, shake, then dry with a towel.

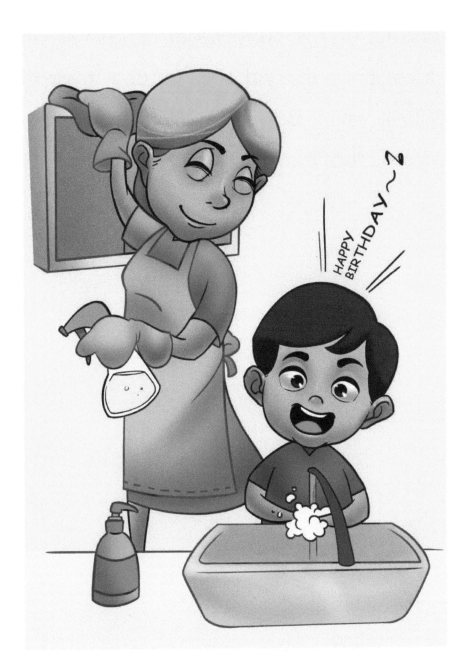

Can I catch it from objects, foods, or plants?

If someone who has the disease sneezes, coughs or wipes their spit or snot on the surfaces of things like doorknobs, furniture, toys, phones, and countertops, their germs will stay there for a while. But the main way people catch this disease is from other humans.

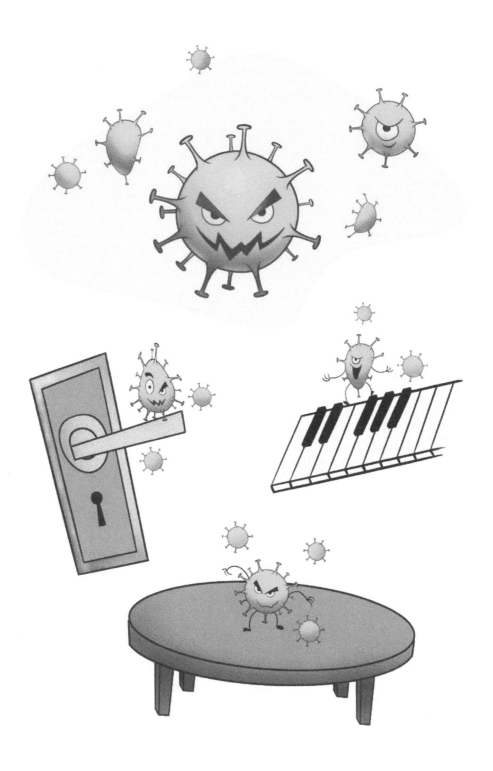

Can I catch it from food?

No. Still, you should always wash your fruits and vegetables before you eat them!

Can I catch it from plants?

No. Plants do get sick, but their sicknesses are very different from ours. Lucky for them, they're safe from this disease.

Can I catch it from pets?

There is a small chance that your pets can infect you, especially if you have cats or ferrets.

If they get sick, ask a veterinarian what to do.

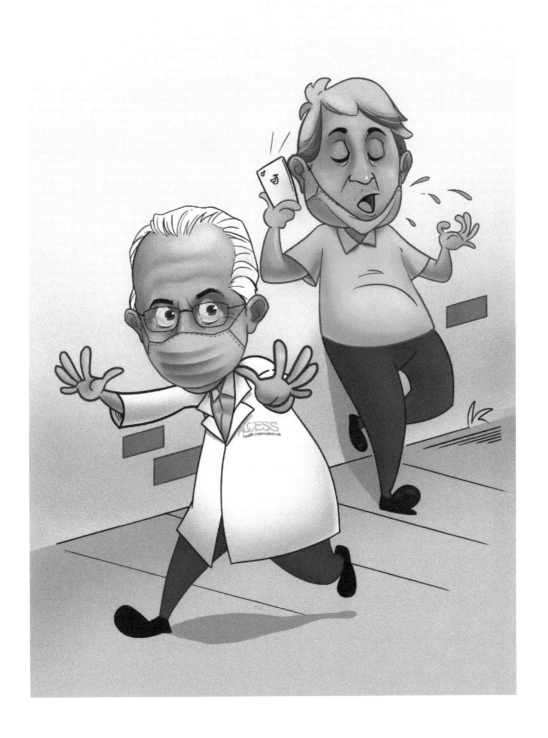

What happens if we catch it?

We don't know. Some people have a little cold. Some people don't feel sick at all.

But for others, like your Grandma and Grandpa, this disease can be very dangerous. Some kids get very sick too.

What if I already have a special disease that other kids don't have?

If you already have a special disease and you get this new disease, there is a greater chance you'll get sick. You and your parents will have to do all the things everyone else is doing to keep themselves safe, like washing your hands often and cleaning the house, but extra carefully.

Remember that all the big changes the world is going through are to protect people just like you. There are many millions of people out there who are staying inside, wearing masks or face shields, and inventing new medicines to try and keep you safe.

If I catch it, will my pets get sick?

Humans can give the disease to animals, so they might.

If you're sick, your parents probably won't allow you to spend much time with your pets. Your pets might even have to stay with someone else for a while. This is to keep them safe.

Is there a medicine that can cure people who get sick, or a vaccine that can keep us from getting sick?

Not yet. Day by day, doctors and nurses are getting better at saving people's lives. When they learn something new about the disease, they quickly tell everybody around the world. It's the same for scientists. They know we're all in this together. There are now some medicines that help people who are very, very sick.

How long will this last? When will it be over?

We don't know for sure. We all hope soon, but it won't be safe to go out until the chances of catching the disease are very low.

Do I have to stay inside the whole time?

As long as the disease is still out there, you'll have to stay inside a lot more than usual.

Being inside so much, there will be times when you—or your parents—feel bored, annoyed, or worried. You might miss your friends or feel sad that so much has changed.

Remember that this is all OK and know that you can always tell a grownup about your feelings. We want you to feel safe, loved, and protected.

What are some fun things I can do if I'm stuck inside all the time?

There is so much you can do to have fun without going outside! You can read a book, paint, do some fun exercises, have a dance party, or watch a movie. You can write letters to your grandparents or play a video game online with friends (as long your parents allow it).

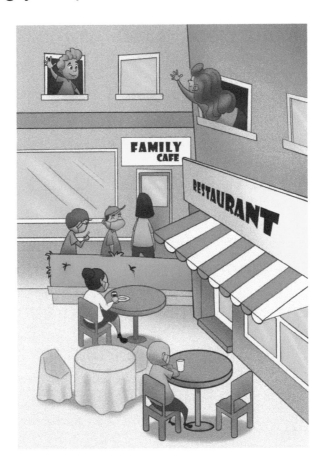

Why are people other than doctors still working? Shouldn't they stay home like me?

Doctors, nurses, and the other people who work in hospitals aren't the only heroes keeping us safe while the disease is still out there.

People working in grocery stores and pharmacies make it possible for us to still have food and medicine. People driving our buses and cleaning our streets make it possible for us to get around safely.

What if one or both of my parents has to go to work and can't stay at home? Can I hug them when they come home?

Some jobs can't be done at home, like working at a hospital or grocery store. You might be worried about your parents if they have jobs like these, but remember they're following extra special rules to keep themselves, and everyone around them, safe.

When they get home, give them space to shower and change into clean clothes since they've been around other people all day. Then you can give them all the hugs you want!

What is the safest way to hug somebody right now?

If you're hugging someone close to your height, make sure you're facing opposite directions.

If you're hugging someone much taller than you, hug them around the knees or waist instead of their neck. You can practice this with your parents!

What if someone outside my family has to take care of me while my parents are working? Am I still safe?

As long as you and the person who is taking care of you still follow the rules that protect us from the disease, like handwashing and social distancing outside, then you'll be as safe as anyone else. That's why they were asked to watch over you—to keep you extra safe.

What happens if one or both of my parents lose their job?

A lot of adults lost their jobs when businesses shut down because of this disease. When a parent loses a job, it can be hard on the whole family.

You might notice that things around your home change a little bit or that your parents are a little more worried than usual. You may feel worried and sad too. That's normal. Don't be afraid to talk to your parents about how you are feeling. Remember, they love you and they will always do their best to take care of you.

If the disease goes away, can it come back?

It might. But by then we may have good ways to protect ourselves if it does.

I'm scared for Grandma and Grandpa. Can I visit them?

It is too dangerous to visit them right now, but you can make them happy by writing them a letter, sending them a card, or calling them on the phone to tell them how much you miss them.

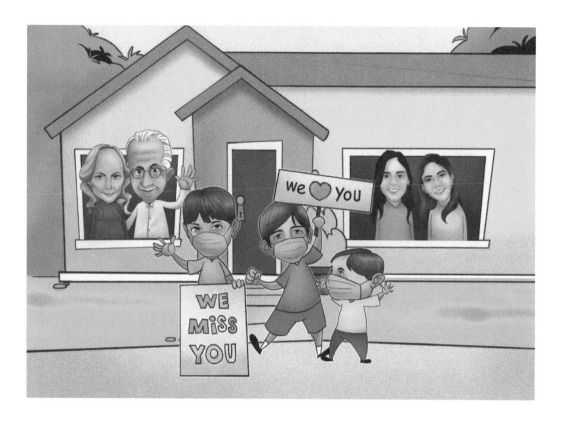

What can I do to help?

You're already helping us stop the disease from spreading by staying home and washing your hands a lot. You're even helping when you cough or sneeze into your elbow instead of all over your hands!

PART TWO

Questions We Ask Ourselves

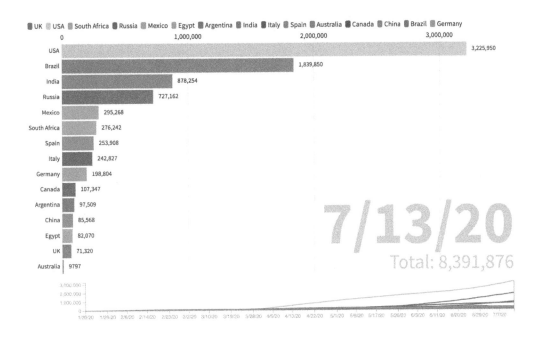

SITUATIONAL AWARENESS

Total number of Covid cases in countries around the world as of July 13, 2020

Source: World Health Organization, July 2020, https://covid19.who.int/

Covid is still a global threat. Until the day that this is no longer the case, we all have a responsibility to stay informed about the dangers this disease presents to our communities, our loved ones, and ourselves. Following certain rules isn't enough to guarantee our safety. We must understand why the rules are there to begin with, and how they change depending on where we are, who we are, and what we're doing.

The first thing we must learn is *situational awareness*. What is the rate of infection in your community, and how likely is it that you're going to encounter someone who is infected?

Start by finding the daily number of new Covid cases in your area at the smallest scale possible—whether it's your county, or your zip code. Using this data, calculate the average number of new cases for the past week. Multiply that number by 10, and you'll have a rough idea of how many people in your community are currently infected.

If the average daily number of new cases is very low—somewhere in the range of 10 to 20—then you can consider yourself relatively safe and free to resume your daily activities. Even though you should continue taking appropriate precautions, you no longer need to isolate at home. If the average daily number of new cases is 50 to 100, you'll need to be more careful. Any number higher than that, and you'll need to be *much* more careful.

In addition to building situational awareness, we must learn to gauge our *personal risk*. Do you have any underlying health conditions that put you at risk? Then you'll need to stay at home as much as possible. A related factor is the *risk of people around you*. Does anyone you're living with have underlying health conditions that put them at risk? If so, your actions will impact them directly.

Whenever you enter a new setting—whether it's your place of work or your child's school—these same factors must be reevaluated, and the risk recalculated. Consider the coworkers on your floor, or the classmates, teachers, janitors, and bus drivers who shuffle in, out, and around the school your child attends. Where are they coming from? What is their risk? If they're at risk, so are you.

Last but not least, we must learn and think critically about the precautions being taken in these settings to keep us safe. Take your child's school. What are they doing to prevent infection, and what will do in the event that infection occurs? Are they conducting temperature screenings? Insisting that students and staff wear masks or face shields? What about social distancing? Don't be afraid to ask questions and, if you're dissatisfied with the answers, advocate for a better solution.

The complex *hierarchy of risk* I describe above can be broken down into the questions below:

1. **How many people are infected on a daily basis in my community?** Remember, multiply by 10 to get a rough estimate of the number of active infections. **Am I or someone in my household at higher risk?**

2. **Will the activity be indoors or outdoors?** The risk is twenty times higher indoors than outdoors.

3. **How long will I be there?** The shorter, the better—especially if the activity is indoors.

4. **How many people will be there?** The fewer, the better.

5. **Will they be wearing masks or face shields?** For an activity to be safe, especially if it's indoors, the answer must be yes.

6. **What precautions are staff, hosts, administrators, or whoever is in charge taking to ensure my safety?**

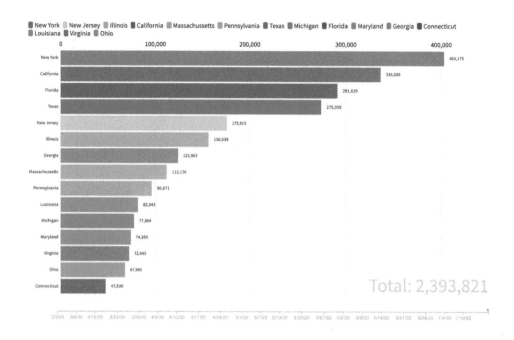

States with highest total number of Covid cases as of July 15, 2020

Source: The COVID Tracking Project, July 2020, https://covidtracking.com/data/download

PROTECTION AND PREVENTION

How do I avoid getting the disease?

By avoiding exposure as much as possible. Stay home when you can, and when going out stay six feet away from the people around you. Wear a mask or face shield when appropriate.

As the country begins to open back up again and people return to work, protecting ourselves will become more difficult. Hence, the hierarchy of risk outlined above.

What if I can't work from home?

Your job may demand that you not only have to spend your day out of the house, but also interact with many people and/or take public transport. If possible, avoid ride sharing and taking public transport at rush hours. Leave accessories like jewelry or watches at home. Keep some hand sanitizer on your person instead, especially if a sink isn't easily within reach at all times.

When coming home, leave your shoes at the front door and toss your dirty clothes into a designated hamper or bag straightaway. (If you have a washing machine at home, throw them in there instead.) If possible, take a shower; if not, wash your hands and change into a clean set of clothes.

For more information on how people with specific occupations can keep themselves safe, consult the guide to worker safety and support compiled by the U.S. Centers for Disease Control and Prevention that is linked at the bottom of the page.[1]

†If I need to take public transport, how do I stay safe?

Before and after, wash your hands.

While riding, stay six feet away from everyone else, keep your mask or face shield on, and avoid touching your face.

---

[1] https://www.cdc.gov/coronavirus/2019-ncov/community/worker-safety-support/index.html

What medical equipment should we have at home to cope with Covid?

The medical devices listed below can be used to accurately monitor your symptoms at home. They are available for purchase at relatively low prices through Amazon and other online retailers.

A thermometer. The best allow you to take someone's temperature without actually touching their skin. A forehead or ear thermometer is best.

A *pulse oximeter.* This measures the amount of oxygen in the blood. This is a simple device that clips onto an index finger.

If the oxygen saturation level reading is below 95 percent, it is time to go to a hospital.

A *defibrillator.* This is used to treat a person who has collapsed because of a heart attack. It is good to have it in the house for family and friends who visit.

A *blood pressure cuff*. Hypertension is one of the major causes of preventable death worldwide.

The defibrillator and blood pressure cuff are not specific for Covid, but I think every household should have them.

†How do I know if a Covid-related product being sold online is real or fake?

Avoid products that are advertised as a cure for Covid-19, or a guarantee of protection from infection. No such thing currently exists. Also pay attention to whether or not the product or its seller has poor ratings or none at all.

Remember to check the drug on several websites. The most reliable are those of the U.S. Food and Drug Administration[2] and the U.S. Centers for Disease Control and Prevention.[3]

---

[2] https://www.fda.gov/consumers/health-fraud-scams/fraudulent-coronavirus-disease-2019-covid-19-products
[3] https://www.cdc.gov/coronavirus/2019-ncov/index.html

When do I wear a mask?

Wear a mask in public settings, particularly in places like airports, grocery stores, and pharmacies where it is difficult to stay six feet away from the people around you.[i] Only children under the age of two and people who already have difficulty breathing shouldn't wear some kind of cloth face cover in these situations.

Evidence shows that throughout the pandemic, mask-wearing has played a crucial role in preventing the spread of disease.[ii] The more people wear cloth face covers in public, the greater the chance that those who have already been infected won't be able to infect others.[iii] For more information on masks, check out the guide compiled by *The New York Times* linked at the bottom of the page.[4]

---

[4] https://www.nytimes.com/2020/04/10/well/live/coronavirus-face-masks-guides-protection-personal-protective-equipment.html?smid=em-share

*Is there a specific type of mask I should use?

There are several. Surgical masks will do the job, but so will a bandana, cloth, or scarf—anything that keeps the tiny droplets that come out of your nose and mouth from reaching other people and surfaces. The U.S. Centers for Disease Control and Prevention released a guide on how to make a mask yourself, which is available on their website.[5]

†What about N95 or KN95 masks?

N95 masks have an exceptional ability to filter out potentially harmful particles, which is why they've become something of a household name. While supply shortages make these airtight, medical grade masks hard to come by, KN95 masks offer a worthy substitute and are available for purchase online.

---

[5] https://www.cdc.gov/coronavirus/2019-ncov/prevent-getting-sick/how-to-make-cloth-face-covering.html

Buyer beware, however—many N95 and KN95 masks have been pulled off their virtual shelves after flunking basic safety tests. Before committing to a purchase of either, make sure it has been approved by the U.S. Food and Drug Administration for importation and sale. That list is linked at the bottom of this page.[6]

†Can I use a face shield instead of a mask?

Under certain circumstances, yes. Some doctors, for example, prefer that you use a face shield during an exam so they can hear and see you better.

If you are indoors with many people, it is best to wear either a mask and goggles or a face shield. A face shield covers more of your face than a mask, keeping droplets away from vulnerable points of entry like your nose, eyes, and mouth.

---

[6] https://www.fda.gov/medical-devices/coronavirus-disease-2019-covid-19-emergency-use-authorizations-medical-devices/personal-protective-equipment-euas

For more information on the do's and don'ts of face shields, check out the comprehensive *Wall Street Journal* guide linked at the bottom of the page.[7]

†If I wear a face shield, should I wear a mask, too?

Expert opinions on this question are mixed, so as of now there is no right answer. Some think face shields alone are enough; others think both should be worn just to be safe.[iv]

Can I get carbon dioxide poisoning (hypercapnia) from wearing a mask?

No. Wearing a mask doesn't reduce the amount of oxygen you're getting. Nor does it increase your level of carbon dioxide. Both oxygen and carbon dioxide are gases that diffuse through masks easily, which is why you can still

---

[7] https://www.wsj.com/articles/what-we-know-about-face-shields-and-coronavirus-11592321931?st=i4dcpazmkmnudz0&reflink=article_email_share

breathe while wearing one, unless you have an underlying lung condition.[v]

Should I wear gloves?

Yes, but wearing gloves can't substitute for handwashing. Remember that if you're out and about, the outside of your gloves can be contaminated. To remove them, you must peel them off from the inside out—and even then, wash your hands afterwards.[vi]

If you're not using disposable gloves, treat them as you would any open surface and clean and disinfect them when you come home.

*Can I continue to take my child to their pediatrician for normal care and vaccinations?

Yes. Children need to have regular checkups, and insofar as it is possible, this care must continue. The same goes for vaccinations. Just because one virus is currently demanding our attention doesn't mean your child is safe from all others.[vii]

The specifics of where, when, and how your appointment takes place will depend on your pediatrician. Call them to learn more.

I am the sole caretaker of my children. What do I do if I need to take them to the grocery store with me?

First, come up with a list of everything you need to buy before you leave. This will save you time you'd otherwise spend aimlessly browsing the aisles. Before you leave, make sure all children over the age of two are wearing masks or face shields.

Once you get to the store, wipe down your cart before you place your baby or child in it. Discourage your kids from touching things and approaching people too closely. They should stay close to you at all times, for their sake and the people around you.

As soon as you're home, both you and your kids should change into clean clothes and throw the dirty ones into the laundry machine or hamper. Shower and bathe if you can. If neither of these options aren't immediately possible, everyone should at least wash their hands.

*Is it safe for me to leave my child at a daycare center or drop them off for an organized group activity?

In the end, decisions about your child returning to daycare or regular group activities should be based on your family's comfort level around the possible risk of infection. If you're worried that your daycare center or childcare program isn't following safety guidelines, don't hesitate to bring it up with staff. Together, you may be able to develop a plan of action and source protective equipment to improve how kids are cared for.

For more information on how childcare programs and daycare centers can keep workers and children safe, check out the guidelines published by the U.S. Centers for Disease Control and Prevention[viii] or the resource for parents created by Child Care Aware[ix].

*In the event of a medical emergency unrelated to Covid, can I still go to the emergency room?

If you're facing a life-threatening emergency, such as a stroke or heart attack, yes. Do not hesitate to call 911 or go to the nearest ER.

Getting immediate medical attention for minor emergencies will be more difficult than usual at this time, as hospitals are currently overwhelmed with Covid patients.

*Can I still go to the dentist?

Unless the infection rates in your community have dipped below 10 to 20 per day, or you have a dental emergency, it is not recommended that you do.[x]

If you must, ask your dentist about the precautions their office is taking to prevent the spread of Covid. If possible, make any necessary changes to your information remotely, so as to minimize your time spent in any common areas. Don't forget to bring your mask or face shield and tight-fitting goggles, too.

Should I still allow workers into my home, like nannies, plumbers, electricians, or cleaners?

If infection rates are high in your community, try to reduce visits from outsiders as much as possible, or avoid them entirely. If you cannot avoid having visitors to your home, make sure you provide them with protective gear upon entry—like masks and hand sanitizer—so they can protect themselves, their families at home, and you.

If it's possible, ask other members of your family to stay in a separate room while they are in your home. If it's not, keep a safe physical distance from the workers while they are in your home and make sure to keep rooms as well ventilated as possible. For some workers, like nannies, this won't be possible. But for cleaners, handymen, and others, it should.

After the visit is over, give your visitor the opportunity to disinfect their hands and any materials they brought into your home. And after they leave, disinfect the areas in your home they visited as well.

How can I care for people who used to work for us regularly but who we can no longer employ because of social distancing restrictions?

These are challenging times for everyone. If you are among those who are able to remain financially stable during these times, consider paying your staff throughout the crisis. A significant loss of income can drive people to make riskier choices, not out of ignorance but out of necessity. If you cannot continue to pay a full salary to any staff, consider offering a smaller amount or offering them an advance on future work.

For those struggling with their own financial worries, providing any form of support may be challenging. In this case, you might want to try connecting former workers with other potential sources of support, like local food banks, loans, or government stimulus support.

I think a friend, family member, or loved one is at risk. What can I do to keep them safe?

If the loved one *isn't* a member of your household, make sure they're in contact with a primary care provider who is familiar with their medical history and can advise them on appropriate precautions to take. Should they start experiencing symptoms—for Covid, or for another serious illness—they must notify their provider as soon as possible and keep them updated on any developments.

You can explore which nearby hospitals offer the highest quality of care and talk to them about where they can go if their condition worsens. Check in with them regularly to see how they're feeling and provide comfort to the best of your abilities. When routine clinical care is not guaranteed, emotional support can be valuable.

These basic guidelines still apply if the loved one *is* a member of your household, but with the added emphasis on creating a safe, clean environment that minimizes any further risk. Use household cleaners and wipes to disinfect the house daily. Wash your hands often, especially after going outside. Know what to do in the event your loved one gets sick and needs some level of home isolation.

*When I'm cleaning and disinfecting my home, how do I know if I'm actually killing the virus?

Experts agree that to eliminate the virus completely, you probably need to spend more time scrubbing down surfaces than you think.[xi] To know just how long you should leave a product on a given surface before toweling it dry, double check the label. It could be as little as 30 seconds, or as much as several minutes.

If you want to verify that a cleaning product is effective against the SARS-2 virus, consult the list compiled by the U.S. Environmental Protection Agency that is linked at the bottom of the page.[8] Remember that ingesting cleaning products or using them to wash yourself or your food can be very harmful.[xii]

---

[8] https://www.epa.gov/pesticide-registration/list-n-disinfectants-use-against-sars-cov-2

How often do I need to wash my bedsheets?

More often than usual. Every time you climb into bed after the end of a long day, you shed sweat, dirt, dead skin—and, if you're infected, bits of SARS-2 virus. While no magic number of washes exists, experts suggest halving the time between wash periods.[xiii] Don't forget to wash or disinfect your laundry hamper as well.

What do I do if I've been exposed to Covid? How long will it be before I'm contagious?

Because Covid is highly infectious, anyone who has been exposed to someone with the disease should consider themselves infected and should isolate themselves from all others.

If you are in fact infected, it could take anywhere three days to three weeks for you to become contagious. According to the World Health Organization, you'll be able to spread the virus to others three to five days before symptoms start to show up.[xiv]

Ideally, your self-isolation would happen at a facility that was monitored and supervised by public health officials.

Realistically, this probably means isolating yourself in a hotel room or in a bedroom in your own home. No one should enter the room that you are in for any reason. Food should be left outside your door; garbage should be collected the same way and immediately disposed of; and— if it is necessary for you to leave the room to go to the bathroom, for example—you should wear a mask or face shield and gloves at all times and ensure the shared room is disinfected immediately after use.

How do I care for someone who is sick with Covid?

If possible, they should be isolated in a hotel room or another location where they can recover. If it does fall to you to take care of someone sick with Covid, the chances you will be infected are extremely high.

If they've consulted a healthcare provider themselves, or if you've consulted a healthcare provider for them (e.g. for your child), you'll need to help them follow any instructions given and pick up any medications prescribed, in addition to suggested over-the-counter medicines. Remember, you may be infected and infectious too, so try to have medications delivered and dropped off at your door.

Make sure they're consuming a lot of fluids, getting a lot of rest, and staying away from pets, if you have any. Monitor and log their symptoms to track any changes for better or for worse. Get in touch with a healthcare provider if you're nervous or unsure about which symptoms are common and which are warning signs.

If I or someone else in my household is infected, will everyone get sick?

The hard truth is that if someone in your household is sick, it will be very hard for you and others in your household to not become infected as well. The ideal situation to protect yourself and the rest of your family is to relocate the sick person to a hotel room or a supervised health facility.

If relocation isn't an option, how do I protect myself and other people in my home if someone gets sick?

Do your best to isolate the person within your home, in a separate bedroom with access to a separate bathroom. Food should be left outside the door of the room and any garbage should be collected in the same way. Silverware and dishes should not be shared under any circumstances and any clothes should be thoroughly washed in hot water immediately.

If the sick person must leave the isolation area to use the bathroom or for another reason, they must wear a mask or face shield and gloves at all times and the shared area should be thoroughly disinfected once the sick person has left.

What if I have small children?

Take the time to plan for back up care should the caregivers in your household fall severely ill.

If your kids are older, involve them in the caregiving process. Give them access to your medical history and the names of your healthcare providers so they can step in and care for you if you yourselves cannot.

†What if I have pets?

If you get sick, there is a chance your pets could catch the disease from you. Cats and ferrets have a higher chance of getting infected than dogs, but we don't have enough information to know which species, if any, are safe.

Find someone who would be willing to take care of your pet(s) in the event you get sick. Otherwise, every time you interact with your pet, you'll have to wear a mask or face shield and wash your hands before and after to try and prevent infection. For more information, watch the short video clip created by the U.S. Food and Drug Administration linked at the bottom of the page.[9]

*How can I manage my Covid-related anxiety?

You can start by moderating your intake of Covid-related news. As important as it is to stay informed, it's also important to recognize when too much is too much. Learn to take a break or walk away when you start to feel

---

[9] https://www.youtube.com/watch?v=KHMYC5Comio&feature=emb_logo

overwhelmed by what you're reading or watching. Impose time limits if necessary.

Engage in some form of physical activity daily and unburden your mind by talking out your worries with family and friends. Schedule a weekly video call with someone to replace your weekly coffee or lunch. Don't forget to be kind to yourself and make time to unwind.

For more information on Covid-related anxiety and ways to cope, check out the *HuffPost* guides linked at the bottom of the page.[10] [11]

How can I help older relatives and neighbors who are living in isolation?

As you would with anyone else who is at risk, check in often and ask what you can do for your relative or neighbor that

---

[10] https://www.huffingtonpost.co.uk/entry/10-sneaky-ways-your-coronavirus-anxiety-is-coming-out_uk_5ec50185c5b6c1f21e70dd93?utm_campaign=share_email&ncid=other_email_o63gt2jcad4&guccounter=1
[11] https://www.huffpost.com/entry/uncertainty-stress-how-to-cope_l_5ed0047cc5b6521c93a80e43?utm_campaign=share_email&ncid=other_email_o63gt2jcad4

might be helpful. Video calls can also take the edge off prolonged isolation.

For more tips and expert advice on how to help older relatives and neighbors, check out the resource created by *The Washington Post* linked below.[12]

What do I do if my parent or spouse or grandparent is in a nursing home?

Check in with them frequently. Ask them about their health, how they feel, and the quality of care they're receiving. Speak with their staff and caregivers, too. Ask them about what they're doing to keep the disease out and what they'll do if it gets in. Request that your loved one's temperature be taken twice daily. If their temperature ever exceeds 100.4 degrees Fahrenheit, insist that they be taken to a hospital immediately.

---

[12] https://www.washingtonpost.com/lifestyle/2020/05/06/seniors-isolation-quarantine-help-how-to/

If, based on conversations with staff and your loved one, you come to the conclusion that they're not safe, it may be time to have a conversation about bringing them home. Both the U.S. Centers for Disease Control and AARP have cautioned against moving older adults out of nursing homes and long term care facilities since the process could unnecessarily expose them to infection.[xv] Even so, the decision should ultimately be made on a case by case basis by the resident and their loved ones.

If my child or relative is living with a disability, how can I protect them from getting sick?

Those who live with mobility impairment, cognitive disability, or any other condition that impedes their ability to follow basic prevention guidelines around social distancing and handwashing are, according to the U.S. Centers for Disease Control and Prevention, at increased risk of getting sick with Covid.[xvi]

To protect them, devise a backup plan for care provision in case their current caregiver gets sick—whether that's you, a home care worker, or someone else. Pull together a network of contacts you or your loved one might reach out to for support that includes neighbors, local service agencies, and friends and family.

Help your loved one stock up on food and medications as much as restrictions allow. Think of other routines that will require rethinking due to lockdown or other Covid-related disruptions and work with your loved one's support network to figure out necessary adjustments.

What if my child or relative is living with a serious mental illness?

This will largely depend on the specific ways in which they feel impacted or vulnerable. For more information, consult the free Covid Resource and Information Guide created by the National Alliance on Mental Illness.[13]

†What if my child or relative uses drugs?

The Harm Reduction Coalition has prepared a resource with guidance for people who use drugs and harm reduction programs and want to stay safe during this pandemic. For more information, as well as translations in Spanish, Portuguese, Arabic, and more, visit the link at the bottom of the page.[14]

TRANSMISSION

†How do I know if I'm at risk?

If you suspect you may be at risk, call a health provider. According to the U.S. Centers for Disease Control and

---

[13] https://www.nami.org/covid-19-guide

[14] https://harmreduction.org/miscellaneous/covid-19-guidance-for-people-who-use-drugs-and-harm-reduction-programs/

Prevention, older adults and people with underlying health conditions are at the greatest risk for severe illness.

Underlying health conditions that have been confirmed to increase risk are:

Chronic kidney disease

COPD (chronic obstructive pulmonary disease)

Immunocompromised state (weakened immune system) from solid organ transplant

Obesity (body mass index [BMI] of 30 or higher)

Serious heart conditions, such as heart failure, coronary artery disease, or cardiomyopathies

Sickle cell disease

Type 2 diabetes mellitus

Underlying health conditions and risk behaviors that are suspected to increase risk are:

Asthma (moderate-to-severe)

Cerebrovascular disease (affects blood vessels and blood supply to the brain)

Cystic fibrosis

Hypertension or high blood pressure

Immunocompromised state (weakened immune system) from blood or bone marrow transplant, immune deficiencies, HIV, use of corticosteroids, or use of other immune weakening medicines

Neurologic conditions, such as dementia

Liver disease

Pregnancy

Pulmonary fibrosis (having damaged or scarred lung tissues)

Smoking

Thalassemia (a type of blood disorder)

Type 1 diabetes mellitus[xvii]

†Does having a certain blood type put me at greater risk of infection or becoming very sick?

Several studies show that those with type A blood have a slightly higher chance being infected and, once infected, seriously ill.[xviii] However, people of all blood types can become seriously ill with Covid.

*Beyond high-risk groups like older adults and those with certain underlying health conditions, does Covid impact some populations more than others?

Yes. Studies clearly show that in the United States, Covid has disproportionately affected minority groups, especially African American, Latino, American Indian, Alaska Native, and Pacific Islander populations.[xix]

African Americans are especially overrepresented, accounting for a third of hospitalized patients despite making up only 18% of the community at large.[xx] A more recent Gallup report included a finding even more startling: that African Americans and Latinos are twice as likely to die from Covid than Caucasians.[xxi]

Similarly, in the United Kingdom, Black and South Asian people were found to be at higher risk than any other race or ethnicity.[xxii]

Why are some populations impacted more than others?

The answer to this question goes well beyond Covid. The disproportionate amount of suffering experienced by minority groups during this pandemic speaks to broader and deeper racial disparities that have affected who receives quality healthcare—and who gets to be healthy—for centuries.

Take high blood pressure, or hypertension, as an example. In many studies, hypertension has been identified as one of the most common comorbidities to occur in Covid patients. In the United States, it also happens to be disproportionately prevalent among African Americans. This is not because of biology, but rather the result of other factors like income, living conditions, level of education, and access to transportation and nutritious food.

While these structural inequities shape our lives and actions each and every day, they become acutely felt in times of crisis. This was true of natural disasters like Hurricane Katrina, and it is true of Covid.

Can I get sick from someone who doesn't look sick?

Yes. You can get the disease from people who look and feel perfectly healthy.

Some people who get infected never develop symptoms, but they're still able to infect others. They are *asymptomatic*.

Some people may infect others when they are in an early stage of their sickness. They haven't developed symptoms yet, but they will. They are *presymptomatic*. According to the World Health Organization, people who have Covid are likely able to infect others one to three days before their symptoms first appear.[xxiii] Asymptomatic and presymptomatic cases make up about four out of every ten infections.[xxiv]

Even people who have mild cases of Covid are able to spread it more easily than other respiratory illnesses. They might not feel or seem very sick, but an unusually large concentration of the virus still builds up in their lungs and nasal passages.

Can I catch it from objects and surfaces?

Transmission through objects is not the main way the virus spreads.[xxv] The main way is through close contact with people who have it.

But in theory, yes. If droplets containing the SARS-2 virus end up on a doorknob, railing, countertop, phone, toilet, or any number of other surfaces, they could stay there for hours or even days.[xxvi] How long they survive depends on the type of material and other extraneous circumstances, like the weather.

Can I catch it from food delivery and packages that come in the mail?

It is unlikely that you would catch the virus from the surface of a package or its contents, according to the U.S. Centers for Disease Control.[xxvii] But packages don't deliver themselves, and it's in the hand-off from the delivery person to the recipient that the greatest risk of transmission lies. The same is true of ordering takeout or a grocery delivery.

To keep yourself and the person handling your delivery safe, make payments online or over the phone when possible and request that deliveries be left outside your house or in the lobby. If you do need to accept a delivery in person, maintain the standard six feet of distance, then wash your hands afterward.

*Can I get sick from airborne transmission?

Yes. The SARS-2 virus, once breathed or sneezed out, can linger in the air as tiny aerosol particles for a few hours.[xxviii] [xxix] This is especially true in closed rooms or airplanes.

When someone sick with Covid coughs, about 3,000 virus-laden droplets fly out of their mouth at a speed of 50 miles per hour. When they sneeze, ten times as many droplets are released at four times the speed.[xxx] Even loud talking releases droplets that can fill a room and stay in the air for several minutes if you're indoors.[xxxi]

The droplets themselves can contain hundreds of millions of virus particles that, once unleashed, flood their surrounding environment. This is why wearing a mask or face shield and covering your mouth and nose when you cough and sneeze is no small matter.

†What is the difference between aerosols and droplets?

Aerosols are droplets, too—they're just very, very tiny.

When we talk about droplets, we're usually referring to the larger ones you expel when you sneeze, cough, or talk loudly. They can land on the surfaces of objects and linger there. Aerosols, on the other hand, are what you release when you breathe or talk normally.

So far, the difference—if any exists—in how droplets and aerosols transmit and spread the virus is unclear.[xxxii]

*Is it easier to transmit the virus indoors?

Yes, the risk of transmission is greater in a closed room than in open air, especially if ventilation is poor and air is stagnant.[xxxiii] Even if you and the other people in the room are wearing masks or face shields, there is bound to be leakage. If one person isn't wearing a mask or face shield, the risk is all the greater.

In this situation, your chances of getting infected yourself depend on how physically close you are to the person and how much time you spend together. Consider the formula below.

Probability of infection indoors = (Time/Distance) * Number of people * Number of people without masks or face shields * % Newly infected in your community

†Can the virus be transmitted through feces or sewage?

Yes. When a virus travels what is known as the *oral fecal route*, it goes from the feces of one infected person into the mouth of another. This could happen at a public pool or a public toilet, by way of contaminated water or sewer gas.[xxxiv] [xxxv]

Does population density affect how the virus is transmitted?

Remember how in the early days of the outbreak, much of our focus was on clusters of cases that broke out in nursing homes, cruise ships, family gatherings, and other conditions of crowdedness and enclosure?

So far, the data amassed on mortality and transmission rates indicate that it is these kinds of cramped environments—within individual homes and buildings—rather than urban environments at large that do more to spread the disease.[xxxvi]

Can children transmit the virus to adults?

Yes. The coronavirus is a member of a family of viruses that cause more than 20 percent of all common colds.[xxxvii] Since we all know that children can transmit colds to adults, there is no reason to think that they would not transmit Covid, too.

Children who are infected with Covid often have very high levels of the virus in their nose and throat, even if they don't have symptoms.[xxxviii]

*How often do animals and humans infect each other?

We know that animals can infect humans, but how often or easily they do is unknown.[xxxix]

We also know that humans can infect animals, which is why people sick with Covid should stay away from their pets. We can be reasonably confident that many species, including household pets like dogs and cats[xl], zoo animals[xli], and farmed mink[xlii], have caught Covid from their human keepers.

We also know that some species are vulnerable because they were infected on purpose for lab experiments, like hamsters and monkeys.[xliii]

GETTING SICK

*If I'm infected, what is the likelihood I'll develop symptoms?

Covid begins as all colds do: with an infection in the upper respiratory tract, nose sinuses, and throat. It can also enter the body through the mouth or intestines if you drink water contaminated with raw sewage.

About two people in every ten who are infected never know it. They have no symptoms—not even a mild cold. They can, however, transmit the virus to others for one to two weeks.

About six people out of every ten have cold symptoms. It may seem like a mild cold, or even a serious one. Some people may have a fever and a cough. Some may lose their sense of smell and taste. Losing your taste and smell is a sure sign of Covid.

The remaining two of every ten who are infected become very ill. People whose infections advance to this stage have described feeling as if a huge weight is on their chest, or like burning tar has been poured into their lungs. They run a high fever above 101.2 degrees Fahrenheit. They are short of breath and feel weak and achy all over. Many can't get enough oxygen and must go to the hospital. Everyone who gets this sick describes it as one of the worst things that has happened to them. Many return to their home, still ill but recovered enough to breathe on their own. It may take a month or two to recover full strength.

Of the 20 percent who need hospitalization, about one in three become so ill that they need to be cared for in an intensive care unit. To stay alive, many need mechanical ventilation to force oxygen into their lungs. They are given powerful drugs that partially paralyze them so they can endure the process. People may remain in intensive care for one or two weeks. Recovery is very slow, as people are weak from the disease and from not moving for a long period.

Covid is sometimes fatal. In the best hospitals, about 1 to 2 percent of people die.

Doctors around the world are learning every day how to care for Covid patients given the tools they have. The good news is that many more people are surviving the most serious effects of the disease now, in mid-2020, than they were at the beginning of the outbreak. But even if symptoms aren't severe, evidence from multiple sources shows that they can last a long time. One survey found that 91 percent of participants had symptoms for 40 days on average.[xliv]

Phases of COVID-19

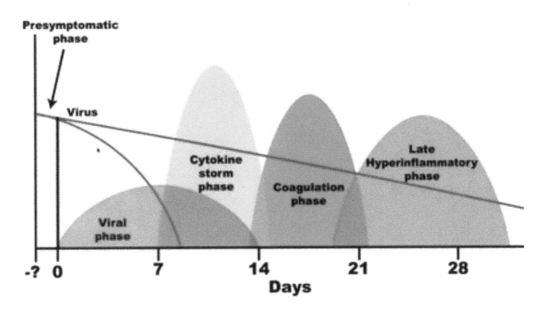

Source: "COVID-19 Testing: How Long Is Someone Infectious Enough To Be Able to Spread The Virus? How to Limit Undetected Infectious Days?", July 2020, https://www.vumedi.com/video/covid-19-testing-how-long-is-someone-infectious-enough-to-be-able-to-spread-the-virus-how-to-limit-u/

*What symptoms should I watch out for?

Check the official website of the U.S. Centers for Disease Control, linked at the bottom of the page, for the most up-to-date information on symptoms.[15] Below is the list available as of this writing:

Fever or chills

Cough

Shortness of breath or difficulty breathing

Fatigue

Muscle or body aches

Headache

New loss of taste or smell

Sore throat

---

[15] https://www.cdc.gov/coronavirus/2019-ncov/symptoms-testing/symptoms.html

Congestion or runny nose

Nausea or vomiting

Diarrhea

What is Covid toe? Is it a symptom?

Covid toe refers to the painful, chilblain-like lesions, either deep red or purple, that have appeared on the toes of some people with mild or otherwise asymptomatic cases of Covid.[xlv]

In children, these toe lesions could also be a symptom of Multisystem Inflammatory Syndrome in Children (MIS-C), otherwise known as Pediatric Multisystem Inflammatory Syndrome (PMIS).

What do I do if I develop symptoms?

Isolate yourself, rest, and call your health provider for further instructions. If you don't have one, call the hotline for Covid at a nearby hospital.

If you share a home with others, chances are they're already infected. If possible, relocate to a hotel room or another location where you can live alone for the duration of your sickness.

*If I'm sick, how long will it take me to recover?

It depends on the severity of your illness. According to the World Health Organization, it usually takes about two weeks from when symptoms first appear for someone with a mild case of Covid to recover. For people with severe cases, it takes longer—anywhere from three to six weeks.[xlvi]

There have been some reports of Covid cases that last even longer.[xlvii]

I'm a single parent. How can I prepare myself in case I get sick?

Stock up on over-the-counter medicines, tissues, and other necessities like nonperishable soups and foods. If you do get sick and develop mild symptoms, such a supply will allow you to recover comfortably at home without needing to go outside.

Have someone in mind who might be able to bring you groceries. Pack a compact overnight bag in case you have a more severe case of Covid and need to go to the hospital.

I'm a single parent. How can I prepare my child in case I get sick?

Reach out to healthy friends, family members, or neighbors who don't belong to a high-risk group and see who would be willing and able to care for your children, even if they're potentially infected or contagious.

Pack a bag for them that includes clothes and a comfort item like a stuffed animal or special blanket, medications, copies of their insurance cards, and a list of names and phone numbers for their pediatricians, teachers and principal, and emergency contacts.

If no one is able to watch your child while you're sick, you'll need to wash your hands regularly, keep your windows open to increase ventilation, and avoid sharing items with them. Whenever you're in the same room, wear a mask or face shield and try your best to keep your distance.

†What are the potential short-term effects of Covid?

Covid can trigger the formation of blood clots. These blood clots travel to the heart, where they can block arteries and potentially lead to a heart attack, or to the brain, which can lead to a stroke. Blood clots can cause damage to the lung and kidneys as well.[xlviii] Many hospitalized patients now receive blood thinners to prevent such clots from forming.[xlix]

†What are the potential long-term effects of Covid?

Many of the long-term effects are still unknown. Those who are sick enough to require ventilation or intensive care may suffer from lifelong injury to their lungs, heart, kidney, and brain. Covid may also induce serious strokes, leading to other forms of long-term disability.

Even those with mild cases of Covid may be diagnosed with chronic disease syndrome (myalgic encephalomyelitis/chronic fatigue syndrome, or ME/CFS), a set of persistent symptoms that can include crushing fatigue, muscle pain, and cognitive problems.[l]

More recent evidence suggests that Covid might be linked to brain damage and diabetes.[li] [lii] About 20 percent of people who end up in the intensive care unit develop neurological complications, some of which can be long-term.[liii]

Can Covid be dangerous for young adults, like it is for older adults?

Covid is dangerous for everyone, from newborns to the very old. People of all ages have died from the infection.

The chance of death from Covid is higher for older people than younger people. Below is a bar graph, sorted by age, of deaths from Covid in New York City. Notice that Covid kills young, middle-aged, and older adults.

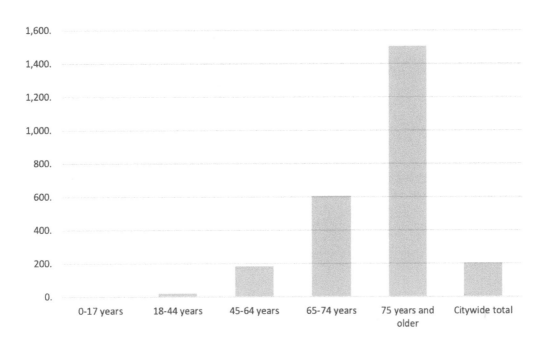

Deaths from COVID-19 in New York City, by age (per 100,000 people)

Source: NYC Health, June 2020, https://www1.nyc.gov/

Below is a graph of hospitalizations, intensive care unit admissions, and fatality rates sorted by age. Notice that Covid causes serious disease in people of all ages.

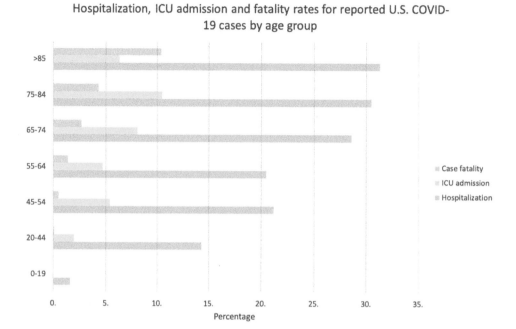

Hospitalization, ICU admission and fatality rates for reported U.S. COVID-19 cases by age group

Source: Statista/Centers for Disease Control and Prevention, March 2020,

https://www.statista.com/chart/21173/hospitalization-icu-admission-and-fatality-rates-for-reported-coronavirus-cases/

Is Covid more dangerous for people who have certain health conditions than others?

Yes. Covid kills more people with other conditions, including people with diabetes, people who are active smokers, people who are overweight (body mass index over 30), people with chronic heart conditions, and people being treated for cancer.[liv] [lv]

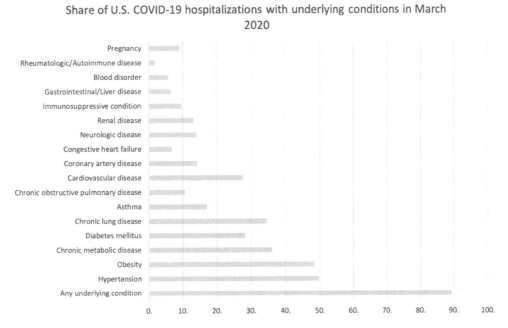

Share of U.S. COVID-19 hospitalizations with underlying conditions in March 2020

Source: MMWR/CDC, April 2020,

https://www.cdc.gov/mmwr/volumes/69/wr/mm6915e3.htm

PREGNANCY AND INFANT CARE

†If I'm pregnant, am I at risk?

As of June 25, pregnant women are now included on the list of at-risk groups maintained by the U.S. Centers for Disease Control and Prevention.

Pregnant women are believed to be at higher risk of developing a serious case of Covid. The disease may also lead to adverse pregnancy outcomes.[lvi]

†If I'm pregnant, what can I do to protect myself and my baby throughout my pregnancy?

More than ever, it is important for you to seek out and keep up your prenatal care plan. Talk to a health provider about creating an appointment schedule and care routines that are right for you and your baby.

In addition to observing more general safety guidelines like social distancing and frequent handwashing, you will need to make an extra effort to limit physical exposure to others, especially strangers.[lvii]

†What if I don't have a health provider?

Contact your local community health center or health department.

†If I'm pregnant and catch Covid, can I infect my baby during pregnancy?

While the answer to this question has for months been unclear, there is some evidence that mothers can transmit the SARS-2 virus to their fetus during pregnancy.[lviii lix lx lxi]

While it may be possible to infect your fetus, as far as we know it is also rare. One of the earliest groups to study the effects of Covid-19 on pregnant women found, out of the nine patients they examined, that none of their newborn children tested positive for the virus.[lxii]

†If I'm pregnant, is it safe to go to a hospital for delivery?

Experts agree that it would be more dangerous for you to give birth at home than at a hospital or certified birth center.[lxiii] While there is a risk that you could become infected with Covid, most hospitals are taking extreme care to separate Covid patients from the rest of their patient population.

†If I'm pregnant, can I infect my baby during childbirth?

Right now, it is unknown whether you can infect the baby during childbirth. However, there is some evidence that you can transmit the virus to your newborn infant, just as you would a cold.[lxiv]

†Can newborn babies be infected with Covid?

Yes. As is the case with many diseases, if a newborn baby becomes infected with Covid, they could become very sick.[lxv] [lxvi]

†After I give birth, am I no longer at risk?

Not necessarily. Because you'll be weakened by labor, and because your newborn will be vulnerable to disease, most experts recommend self-isolating with your baby and anyone else in your household for at least two weeks after giving birth.[lxvii]

†If I get sick, can I continue to breastfeed my child?

Yes. No studies have shown that the virus can be transmitted through breastmilk.

†When can my newborn baby meet their grandparents?

Experts tend to agree that for at least two weeks after giving birth, the mother, newborn child, and anyone else sharing their household should self-isolate. Grandparents who plan on visiting should self-isolate during this period, too, just to be safe.

If, after two weeks of isolation have gone by, all parties are healthy and without symptoms—baby included—their grandparents should be in the clear to make the trip to see their newborn grandchild. If that trip doesn't involve air travel, hotels, or any detours that might expose them to the virus, it might even be possible to hold their grandchild.

For more advice, check out the guide created by *The New York Times* specifically for new moms faced with this problem.[16]

†How can I cope with the stress of being a new mother or mother-to-be in the time of Covid?

Even when a pandemic isn't going on, new mothers and mothers-to-be undergo a turbulent range of emotions— some of which are symptomatic of conditions like perinatal mood and anxiety disorders (PMADs) and postpartum depression. The fear and looming threat of Covid only intensifies an already stressful situation.[lxviii]

Many resources are out there that can help you cope, some of which are linked at the bottom of the page. The March of Dimes has added a special section on "Coping with Stress and Anxiety during the Covid Pandemic" to their free

---

[16] https://www.nytimes.com/2020/06/16/parenting/baby/grandparents-meet-newborn-coronavirus.html

Navigating Your Pregnancy guide.[17] Caring Communities has also released a wellness guide for pregnant mothers that includes its own list of resources[18], while the Maternal Mental Health Leadership Alliance has created an entire directory.[19]

COVID AND CHILDREN

How do I know if my child is infected with the Covid virus?

If your child has developed cold symptoms and you think it might be Covid, call a doctor, preferably one who already knows your child's medical history. Schedule a telehealth visit if possible so your child can be examined without leaving your home. Make sure the child is resting and getting enough fluids.

---

[17] https://www.marchofdimes.org/it-starts-with-mom/coping-with-stress-and-anxiety-during-the-covid-19-pandemic.aspx

[18] https://med.emory.edu/departments/psychiatry/_documents/tips.pregnant.mothers.pdf

[19] https://www.mmhla.org/covid-19/

For the most up-to-date list of Covid symptoms, visit the U.S. Centers for Disease Control and Prevention website linked at the bottom of the page.[20]

What is Multisystem Inflammatory Syndrome in Children (MIS-C)? Should I be afraid that my child will get it?

In some young people, Covid has caused a rare but serious disease called Multisystem Inflammatory Syndrome in Children (MIS-C), otherwise known as Pediatric Multisystem Inflammatory Syndrome (PMIS).

When children develop MIS-C, their blood vessels become inflamed. Symptoms include persistent fever, serious rashes, "strawberry" tongue, bright red toes and fingers, and other inflammatory symptoms.[lxix] If your child has any of the

---

[20] https://www.cdc.gov/coronavirus/2019-ncov/symptoms-testing/symptoms.html

MIS-C symptoms, take them to an emergency room immediately or call 911.

†What are the long-term effects of MIS-C?

One study showed that four out of four children who were admitted to a hospital and diagnosed with MIS-C sustained brain damage. Symptoms included confusion, tremendous fatigue, and impaired coordination.[lxx]

*Besides MIS-C, are there Covid symptoms children have that adults don't?

What usually distinguishes the Covid cases in children from those of adults aren't specific symptoms, but a relative lack of symptoms altogether. Although multiple studies have confirmed that children are capable of transmitting the virus, they usually don't get very sick from it.

There are exceptions. A recent study of five children who were hospitalized and later diagnosed with Covid revealed that all five had problems with their digestive tract (usually diarrhea) that preceded all other related symptoms.[lxxi] This suggests that symptoms like diarrhea and stomach pain might indicate otherwise undetectable cases of Covid.

IMMUNITY

†What does immune system do to help us recover from Covid?

Your immune system works to eliminate the virus. Your body develops antibodies, which bind to and move the virus, and T cells, which recognize and destroy virus-infected cells.

†What are antibodies?

Antibodies are proteins that bind to and help destroy a virus.

*If I recover from Covid, is there still a chance I can infect other people? When can I go out again?

We still don't know enough to say.

Around two weeks after recovery, when the chances of infecting another person are very low, consider getting tested for the Covid virus. If you test negative, you may be in the clear. There have been exceptions, however.

Still: even if you feel fully recovered and your symptoms have disappeared, you should continue to observe protection guidelines as if you'd never gotten sick in the first place.[lxxii]

*If I recover from Covid, am I immune? How long will my immunity last?

Most people who get sick with Covid develop antibodies, and some of these antibodies can fight and neutralize the virus. [lxxiii]

More recent evidence, however, suggests that all these antibodies might fade relatively quickly. If this virus behaves like coronaviruses we've studied before, most people won't be protected for more than a year—leaving the body vulnerable to reinfection from the same virus. [lxxiv lxxv]

Even after you recover, you should take the same precautions as someone who hasn't yet fallen ill. There is a small chance that you can still infect others even after your symptoms have disappeared.

*If I recover from sickness, can I get infected again?

Possibly. There are several reports of reinfection, though none have been confirmed. Reinfection does occur with cold-causing coronaviruses.[lxxvi] [lxxvii]

Should I catch Covid on purpose so I develop immunity to it?

No. We know too little about how immunity against Covid works to assume that contracting the virus leads to prolonged protection from it. Such behavior is dangerous not just for you, but for the people around you.[lxxviii]

†Is it possible for the world to develop herd immunity to Covid?

Probably not. Research on the decline of Covid antibodies, as well as a wealth of studies on the coronavirus family at large, suggests that immunity to these viruses fades too quickly.[lxxix]

PUBLIC HEALTH MEASURES

What is "flattening the curve"?

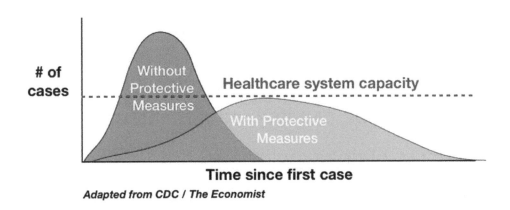

Adapted from CDC / The Economist

Source: Drew Harris/New York Times, March 2020, https://www.nytimes.com/article/flatten-curve-coronavirus.html

Flattening the curve is shorthand for slowing down the rate of transmission. As a strategy, it involves measures like social distancing, self-isolation, and frequent handwashing.

The principal aim of flattening the curve is to keep hospitals from being overloaded. It doesn't necessarily mean reducing the total number of infections, which requires a more aggressive approach: crushing the curve.

To only partially restrict transmission, as some countries have done, is a strategy I call "climbing the mesa." Per this logic, the steep slope of initial rates of infection flattens into a long, bumpy plateau, with the drop-off in new cases somewhere in the distant future. Rates of infection may be reduced from what they first were but remain high for a long period of time.

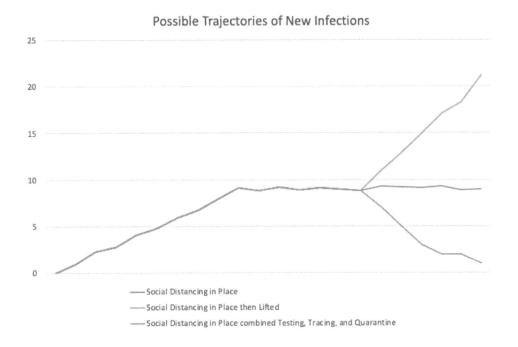

Then there is the mountain beyond the plateau—the third and most dangerous outcome that describes what is happening in countries like the United States. In this scenario, a country is thought to be riding out a mesa, only to discover it is actually at the foot of a mountain.

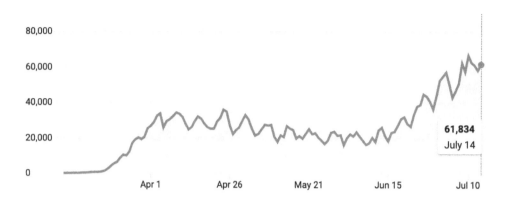

Source: Wikipedia

What is contact tracing?

Contact tracing is a strategy for slowing the spread of Covid infections that involves tracing and monitoring the contacts of people who have been infected—which is to say, those that might have been exposed. Trained volunteers and public health workers work with Covid patients to help them identify these contacts, then work with the contacts themselves to arrange a safe two-week quarantine.

Contact tracing efforts can be assisted by mobile technologies, digital surveillance systems, and private-public partnerships, all of which have been used to varying degrees in countries like South Korea, Taiwan, and China.[lxxx lxxxi]

†What is quarantine? How is it different from isolation?

According to the U.S. Centers for Disease Prevention and Control:

> ***Isolation*** *separates sick people with a contagious disease from people who are not sick.*

> ***Quarantine*** *separates and restricts the movement of people who were exposed to a contagious disease to see if they become sick.*[lxxxii]

Everyone who knows or suspects that they were exposed to Covid-19 should quarantine themselves for at least two weeks.

Everyone who then develops symptoms must isolate themselves until they are two weeks out of recovery.

*When should I get tested?

If you have Covid symptoms and want to get tested, call your health provider. They can instruct you on next steps.

*Where can I get tested?

The availability of testing is largely regional. On the whole, tests are becoming more widely available. In some places, your health provider might have tests on hand. In others, walk-in health clinics could have a supply also. In others still, state and local health authorities may be in charge or organizing testing sites and distributing tests.

For up-to-date information on where you can get tested, visit the website of your state or local health department.

What kinds of tests are available for Covid?

Three types of tests have been approved by the U.S. Food and Drug Administration: RNA tests, which measure the presence of the actual virus; antigen tests, which measure the presence of viral proteins; and antibody tests, which measure the body's reaction to the virus.[lxxxiii]

What are RNA tests and how do they work?

Of the three different types, RNA tests, also known as genome or nucleic acid tests, are useful for detecting active infections. They're the most sensitive and reliable of available Covid tests, but their results also take the most time to deliver—from one day to a week and a half, depending on the context.

RNA tests measure the presence of viral genes in the body using a swabbed sample, usually taken from the nose and throat. The sample must then be sent to a lab where it can be replicated and analyzed in a special machine. The test itself may not take long to complete, but most labs have accumulated a backlog of samples in need of processing that prolongs turnaround time.[lxxxiv]

Point-of-care RNA tests have also been developed that shorten this waiting period to mere minutes, though the World Health Organization recommends limiting use of these tests to research settings only due to a lack of supportive evidence.[lxxxv]

What are antigen tests and how do they work?

While RNA tests detect the presence of viral genes, antigen tests do the same for viral proteins, meaning they can also detect active infections. They are the latest of the Covid tests to be approved by the U.S. Food and Drug Administration, they are also the fastest, though not the most sensitive.

The U.S. Food and Drug Administration cautions that those who test negative for Covid using an antigen test may need to confirm their results with a genome test, or risk acting on a false negative.[lxxxvi] But in addition to yielding fast results, antigen tests are cheaper to produce and easier to scale up to the levels needed to test entire states and nations.[lxxxvii]

What are antibody tests and how do they work?

An antibody test, or serology test, measures the presence of antibodies in the blood, meaning they're good at detecting past infections rather than active infections. Antibody tests are designed to reveal whether or not someone has developed an immune response to the SARS-2 virus, though testing positive doesn't necessarily ensure immunity.[lxxxviii]

Like antigen tests or point of care RNA tests, antibody tests are a rapid diagnostic test that will give users a verdict within minutes. However, their speed and convenience can come at a cost; some users have reported incidents of inaccuracy or trouble interpreting the results in the first place.[lxxxix]

While reports of their inaccuracy have been a cause for doubt, newly licensed versions show promise to be more specific than many already brought to market.

*Are home tests available?

Yes. The U.S. Food and Drug Administration has approved a handful of tests that allow users to collect their own viral samples at home and send them to labs for processing.[xc]

Some companies claim that their at-home tests can deliver results without involving third parties like labs. The U.S. Food and Drug Administration has issued their manufacturers warning letters that effectively declare these claims to be false.[xci] To learn more about which at-home tests have been flagged as fraudulent or misleading, visit the FDA website linked at the bottom of the page.[21]

What about temperature checks?

So-called "fever detectors" and thermal scanners alone cannot reliably identify people who are sick with Covid. These technologies, which claim to pick up on elevated temperatures by measuring the heat coming off a person's skin, have a hard time distinguishing between fevers and other forms of excess body heat.[xcii]

According to one study, screening strategies like airport temperature checks are estimated to miss more than half of infections.[xciii] This isn't exactly surprising, given that many people who have Covid don't even run a temperature.

---

[21] https://www.fda.gov/consumers/health-fraud-scams/fraudulent-coronavirus-disease-2019-covid-19-products

How many tests do we really need?

Ideally, all 155 million workers in the United States should be tested before returning or continuing to work. All 80 million students (kindergarten through grade 12 and college) should be tested before returning to classrooms, which are ideal settings for disease transmission. All those over the age of 65 (about 50 million) should be tested, as they are at high risk.

REOPENING SAFELY

*If my boss wants me to go back to work, what can I do to keep myself and others safe?

If you are healthy and commute to work via public transit, wear gloves to help you avoid getting the virus on your hands. Do not touch your eyes, nose, or mouth, and leave your phone in your pocket throughout your commute to avoid transferring germs onto its surface. If you can, consider taking a bike or car to work instead, being careful to wipe down all surfaces with disinfectant sheets prior to touching any surface.

If you have another medical condition that puts you at high risk for a severe case of Covid, ask your employer to provide you with reasonable low-cost solutions to make the office space safer for you.

This could include moving your work area away from others, limiting foot traffic around your workspace, or using plexiglass, tables or other barriers to ensure a minimum distance between you and your coworkers. You may also want to ask your employer for a change in hours to help you avoid rush hour commutes and to limit the number of employees around you at the office.

If you are sick with a fever or cough—no matter whether you were officially tested and diagnosed with Covid—do not return to the workplace until at least 14 days, ideally up to 16 days, since the onset of your symptoms.

When you do return to work, wear a mask or face shield, keep a safe distance from your colleagues, and be conscious of what you touch in common areas, wiping down surfaces after you touch them.

If you are not sick but someone in your household is showing signs of Covid, do not go into work until your entire household has recovered.

When cities begin to reopen, and I begin to go outside again, how can I keep myself safe?

Assume that everyone is infected and act accordingly.

Continue wearing a mask or face shield, maintaining six feet of distance from the people around you, and washing your hands after going outside. Because subsequent waves of infection, if they occur, will likely spread undetected before the number of confirmed cases begins to surge, it is best to proceed with the utmost caution in the uncertain weeks and months that lie ahead.

To stay safe, we should remember the places and events that proved to be significant sources of transmission in the early days of the outbreak. Large gatherings like birthday parties, weddings, and funerals were what the U.S. Centers for Disease Control and Prevention calls *super-spreading events*. This means that some clusters of Covid cases were traced back to a single social gathering.[xciv] Conferences and networking events held in February were another culprit.

When cities begin to reopen, which places should I avoid? *

Steer clear of buildings and spaces that are confined, poorly ventilated, and densely populated.[xcv] This has less to do with the type of establishment—office, restaurant, what have you—and more to do with the type of environment. If a place you usually frequent has problems with volume and airflow, consider delaying your return or discussing your safety concerns with someone who can address them.

This also applies to places indoors and outdoors where people tend to loosely gather and hang around for extended periods of time—"talking, singing, and panting," as one *Forbes* columnist put it.[xcvi] Such activities tend to promote a general lingering and commingling of particles in the air.

Will it be safe for me to host or take part in small gatherings?

Look to community infection rates, not those of your peer group, when making this decision. If community infection rates haven't yet dropped to single digits or zero, it is safest to gather outdoors at six feet apart and with masks or face shields on.

Recall the following equation:

Probability of infection indoors = (Time/Distance) * Number of people * Number of people without masks or face shields * % Newly infected in your community

*Which outdoor activities are safe for me and my family?

Most outdoor activities are safe if you keep your distance from other people, don't travel too far, and limit outings to you and your household only.[xcvii] That rules out team and contact sports but leaves plenty of room for other kinds of recreation. The U.S. Centers for Disease Control and Prevention also advises us to stay away from crowded parks and playgrounds.[xcviii]

The California state government has compiled a list of safe activities that includes picnicking, watching the sunset, and hiking, so long as the trails are spacious enough to permit six feet of distance.[xcix] Social distancing guidelines apply to runners and bikers, too.

When can I start to spend time with my grandchildren again?

It will be safe to be with your grandchildren again when the chance of contracting Covid in your community is very low. You will know that when, for the previous two weeks, between zero to five people are diagnosed.

A community may be your city, or for those living in smaller towns and communities, your county.

Travel

When will it be safe for me to travel to my non-primary residence?

There is no easy answer to this question because the restrictions and risks involved vary from place to place. Many city and local officials have urged non-primary homeowners to remain in place for the sake of slowing the spread, but as regions reopen and restrictions begin to ease up, the decision will ultimately be left to the individual.

If you're considering relocating to a non-primary residence, consult the websites of the local police department, sheriff's office, and health authorities both of your current location and of your destination to make sure you're not violating any protective guidelines. Make phone calls if necessary.

If I'm driving a long distance, is it safe to stay at hotels or rental properties along the way?

Driving in your own car is safe. Staying overnight in a hotel or rented apartment is much riskier. You can never be sure who was there before you and how well the place was cleaned.

Until the number of new infections at all points of your destination is very low—between zero to five per day—I do not advise traveling unless it is absolutely necessary.

If I'm traveling a great distance by car, which public restrooms are safe for me to use?

While some places are taking precautions like setting up portable toilets, roping off some sinks, or sanitizing their restrooms every half hour, there isn't a way to ensure that a public restroom remains virus-free. If you do need to use a public restroom, keep your mask or face shield on, use a paper towel when touching any surfaces, and of course give your hands a good wash on your way out.[c]

*I need to travel by plane for emergency reasons. What precautions should I take?

It is very difficult to guarantee your safety on a plane. At least for now, there is no guarantee as to how you will be seated and how clean the plane will be.

If you must travel by plane, keep your mask or face shield on at all times as long as you're in the airport. If you're wearing a mask, a TSA official might ask you to lower it when you go through a security checkpoint. Otherwise, keep it on. Shopping or eating at airport restaurants isn't advised. Bring your own food, books, and eye drops instead.

Once on the plane, keep your mask or face shield on as much as possible. Wipe your seat down with disinfecting wipes before you sit in it.

VACCINES AND TREATMENTS

Why don't we have a vaccine yet?

There is good reason why it usually takes several years to make a safe, effective vaccine. The interactions between one virus and the human immune system are very complex. Many viruses have learned to evade our immune defenses.

More than 100 Covid vaccines are currently in development worldwide.[ci] But even if one of these proves effective, it will be at least another year before it is ready and available to all.

Is it possible to speed up vaccine development?

It is possible to speed up the testing of vaccines. Vaccines are given to healthy people to prevent them from becoming sick.

But if the plan is to vaccinate two or three billion people or more, any vaccine must be safe beyond doubt. Up until now, the fastest we have ever produced a vaccine, proven it safe, and made it available for so many people is four years. We might be able to make that timeline a little shorter.

Could a vaccine turn out to be harmful?

Yes. That is why each vaccine candidate must be tested for safety in many people before it can be used to protect what might be billions of people.

This is especially a concern for older adults, who are among the most vulnerable to infection. As we age, our immune system weakens and does not respond as effectively to vaccines as it does when we're young. But some people older than 65 can still be protected by some vaccines, such as the seasonal influenza vaccines.[cii]

Once there is a vaccine, will everybody be able to get it?

Initial batches will likely go to healthcare workers, critically ill patients, and those at highest risk.[ciii] Only then will the vaccine become available for mass use. Billions of doses will need to be manufactured and distributed fairly around the world. How long it takes to vaccinate everyone depends on many factors, cooperation across borders not least among them.

It is very likely that rich countries will get the vaccine before poorer countries. That is unfortunate. I hope this time, things will change. Remember that as long as one person in the world has it, we are all at risk.

How long will it take to make enough vaccine doses for the entire world?

Manufacturing can be a bottleneck. It depends on the type of vaccine. Some are easy to make, some very hard. The good news is that a number of vaccines are given to all children before the age of five and often earlier.

Manufacturing vaccines for the whole world is a challenge we can meet.

†Why don't we have a drug treatment yet?

While drug development generally proceeds at a faster pace than vaccines, it is still important to prioritize safety over speed.

With more than 150 anti-Covid drugs in the running, there is reason to hope that a treatment will emerge within the year.[civ]

*What kinds of drugs are being developed to treat Covid?

Some treatments improve our immunity to the virus and are hence called *passive immune therapies*. These treatments usually involve giving COVID patients protective antibodies that are naturally occurring or manmade.

Another category of treatments attacks the virus itself and prevents it from replicating inside the body. These *antiviral drugs* are designed to counteract the specific ways in which the virus hijacks our cells.

Then there are *immune drugs*, which prevent the immune system from overreacting to the virus and overwhelming other bodily systems. This overreaction is one reason why some people get so sick from COVID.

Monoclonal antibody drugs are made using a single cell that produces a single, highly neutralizing antibody, which is replicated over and over again at a large scale. They have the purity and consistency of a synthetic product, but remain wholly human and, in some cases, very effective. Unfortunately, they can be expensive and difficult to make.

Why are old drugs being tested as potential Covid treatments?

Repurposing either one drug or a combination of drugs can sometimes prove effective in treating a new disease. This was the case for hepatitis C and HIV.[cv]

Can the antibodies of recovered patients be used to treat Covid?

The antibody-rich blood plasma of recovered patients, also known as convalescent sera, has been used to treat emerging infectious disease since the nineteenth century.

Some studies of this experimental therapy, which was also used during the SARS epidemic, have shown reductions in mortality and viral load.[cvi]

In March, the U.S. Food and Drug Administration authorized this approach for emergency use in critically ill Covid patients.[cvii] Use is limited due to the worry that rogue substances in plasma donations could lead to other kinds of infections, especially in patients whose lungs or immune systems are already weak or compromised.

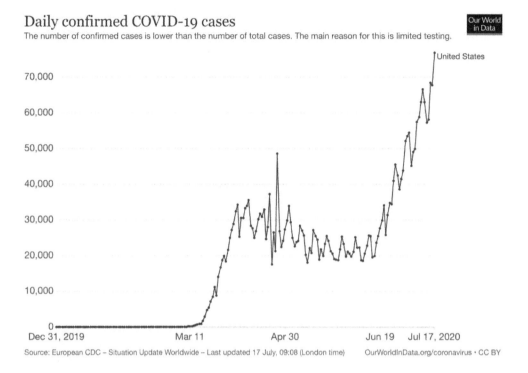

Daily confirmed COVID-19 cases
The number of confirmed cases is lower than the number of total cases. The main reason for this is limited testing.

Source: European CDC – Situation Update Worldwide – Last updated 17 July, 09:08 (London time)   OurWorldInData.org/coronavirus • CC BY

Source: European CDC, July 2020,

https://ourworldindata.org/

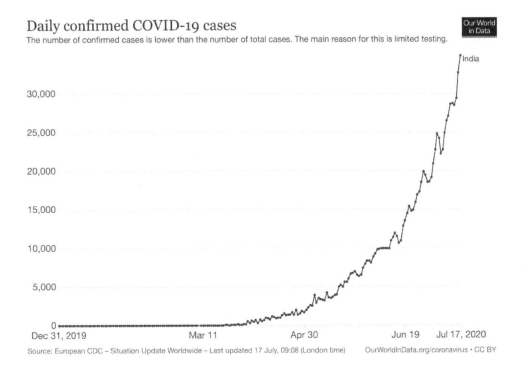

Source: European CDC, July 2020,

https://ourworldindata.org/

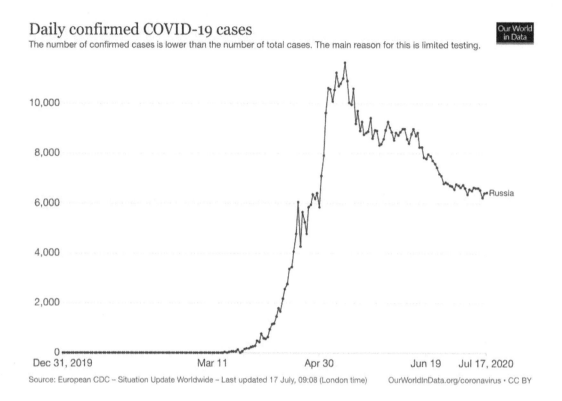

Daily confirmed COVID-19 cases
The number of confirmed cases is lower than the number of total cases. The main reason for this is limited testing.

Source: European CDC – Situation Update Worldwide – Last updated 17 July, 09:08 (London time)   OurWorldInData.org/coronavirus • CC BY

Source: European CDC, July 2020,

https://ourworldindata.org/

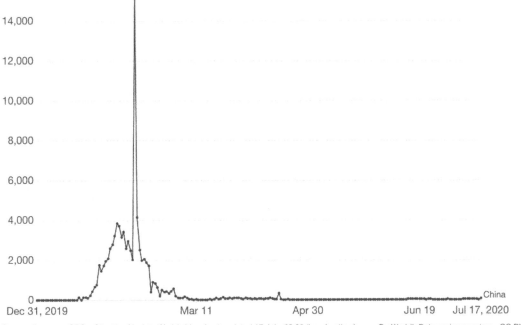

Source: European CDC, July 2020,

https://ourworldindata.org/

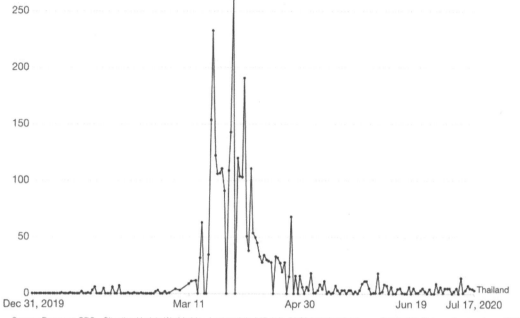

Daily confirmed COVID-19 cases

The number of confirmed cases is lower than the number of total cases. The main reason for this is limited testing.

Source: European CDC – Situation Update Worldwide – Last updated 17 July, 09:08 (London time)   OurWorldInData.org/coronavirus • CC BY

Source: European CDC, July 2020,

https://ourworldindata.org/

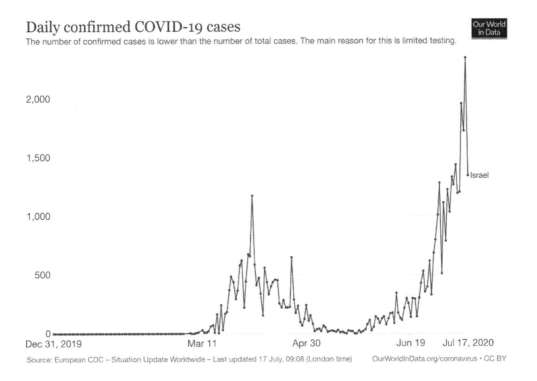

Source: European CDC, July 2020,

https://ourworldindata.org/

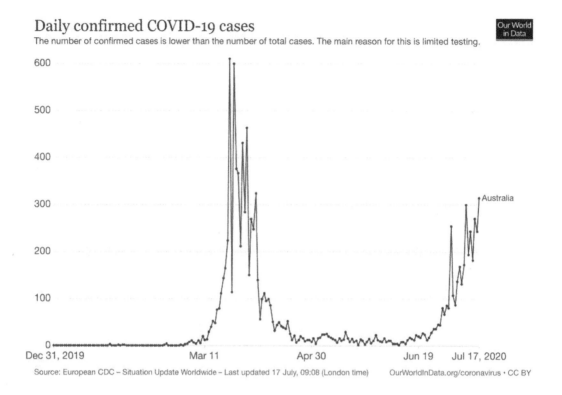

Source: European CDC, July 2020,

https://ourworldindata.org/

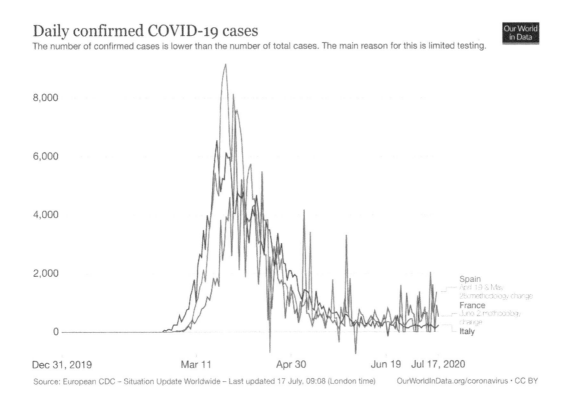

Daily confirmed COVID-19 cases
The number of confirmed cases is lower than the number of total cases. The main reason for this is limited testing.

Source: European CDC – Situation Update Worldwide – Last updated 17 July, 09:08 (London time)   OurWorldInData.org/coronavirus · CC BY

Source*: European CDC, July 2020,*

https://ourworldindata.org/

WHAT DOES THE FUTURE LOOK LIKE?

Will warm weather weaken the disease?

Coronavirus infections that cause colds peak in the winter months. That is why there is hope that infections will slow in the summer. However, we know that some coronaviruses that peak in wintertime persist all year long, albeit at lower levels in the summer months and in the tropics.

MERS, the lethal coronavirus that camels give to humans, occurs in the dry heat of the Middle East. Covid itself is as serious a threat in the hot, humid cities of Singapore and Southern China as anywhere else.

The general consensus is that Covid cases may slow in the summer, but may pick again in the winter months.[cviii]

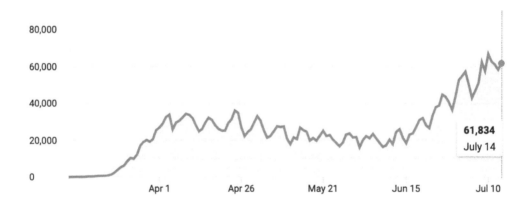

Source: Wikipedia

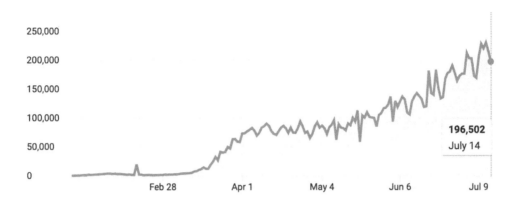

Source: Wikipedia

*Can the virus evolve to become more lethal and more transmissible?

Yes. It has already become more transmissible. The current strain in circulation is ten times as transmissible as earlier strains.[cix]

There is a chance the current strain could become more lethal, even though current evidence doesn't suggest that it has yet. MERS, the last coronavirus epidemic, was caused by a virus more lethal than that which caused SARS, the first.[cx]

Can another coronavirus pandemic occur?

Yes, another coronavirus pandemic is possible and indeed very likely. Covid is the third coronavirus epidemic to occur in the last two decades, the first and second being SARS and MERS, respectively. In the case of all three, the virus originated from bats, but came to infect humans by infecting another mammal first.

For the SARS virus, that mammal was the civet cat. For the MERS virus, it was the camel. For the SARS-2 virus, it remains unknown, though like SARS, it originated from bats found in the caves of southern China.[cxi]

No matter the path from animals to humans, the fact remains that this particular strain—more deadly, and more easily spread, than those that came before—ultimately began with *one person*. Before Covid was a global pandemic, it was one person with a cold. If this happened three times, it could happen again.

It seems like many new infectious diseases have emerged in the last decade. Is that true?

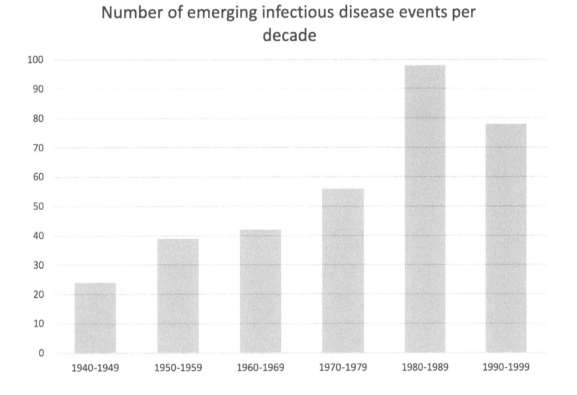

Number of emerging infectious disease events per decade

Source: Jones, K., Patel, N., Levy, M. *et al.* Global trends in emerging infectious diseases. *Nature* 451, 990–993 (2008). https://doi.org/10.1038/nature06536

Yes. Over the last 20 years we have seen many new diseases, especially many new infectious disease outbreaks. This is in large part because of the way humans behave, rather than any change in the number of diseases that exist in nature. A rapid growth in global population, increased urbanization—with more of us crowded together in a smaller geographic space—and increases in travel, trade, and connectivity are the main causes.

What's more, a warming climate means that diseases carried by mosquitoes are moving from the tropics to what used to be colder climates.

Notably, most of these new diseases came from animals. There were the two previous coronavirus epidemics, SARS and MERS, which both originated in bats and then passed to humans through civets. Ebola came from gorillas and chimpanzees; Zika comes from mosquitoes; hantavirus pulmonary syndrome from rodents; and HIV/AIDS originated in chimpanzees.[cxii]

*Will schools reopen in the fall?

The answer to this question varies from place to place, and even from school district to school district. Only when the level of new cases in a community is either very low—less than ten cases per day for a large city—should schools reopen.

Many people think that children aren't easily infected, which isn't actually the case. Young children may not fall ill as often as adults, but that doesn't mean they can't become very sick or spread the disease far and wide. Plus, kids older than the age of 10 have the same chance of being infected as young adults.

Be on the lookout for the supplement I'm currently writing about this topic.

Will school shutdowns affect the mental health of our children?

The world, as our children knew it, has grown very small over the course of the pandemic—and as it opens back up to them, it won't be the same as before. Some will be grieving great losses, others will be struggling with anxiety, disappointment, and disillusionment, and others still will be emerging from a volatile or violent home environment.[cxiii]

So long as these struggles play out within the confines of individual homes, it will be difficult to gauge just how detrimental this has been to the mental health of children across the country.

*Will school shutdowns caused by Covid change the education system for good?

How our children learn will change. Current experiments with remote learning, some of which are based largely on trial-and-error, will evolve into mainstay digital learning tools and modes of instruction. This much is certain.

Also certain is the fact these effects will be variable and uneven, determined in large part by existing gaps in the quality and capabilities of our school systems. The children more likely to benefit from this transition, and even prefer it, are those who already have their own electronic devices and a high-speed internet connection.[cxiv]

Who will these changes impact most?

Children living in low-income and otherwise underserved communities, on the other hand, are currently having a more difficult experience with remote learning. Already they have less access to their virtual classrooms and teachers and spend less time studying overall.[cxv] A similar split can be seen between the students of public and private schools.

As more data on long-term effects emerges, so will opportunities for interventions that level a very unequal playing field for our young learners whose education was interrupted by the pandemic. If not, the gaps will only continue to grow.

*How can colleges and universities reopen safely?

Students should expect reopening strategies to vary. What a large public university does to prevent infection among students, for instance, will likely differ from a citywide community college or small liberal arts college. This applies to questions of on-campus housing, study abroad opportunities, research facilities, and other features of higher education.

The Chronicle of Higher Education has compiled an at-a-glance guide to the reopening strategies of different universities. To compare them, follow the link at the bottom of the page.[22]

How can countries reopen safely?

All public health authorities agree that to reopen a country, region, or state, at least three conditions must be met.

First, the transmission rate has to be very low throughout the entire region—at the highest, five per day. Second, there must be a rigorous testing regime in place to identify who is actually infected. Third, there must be contact tracing and a strategy for isolating those exposed for up to fourteen days or longer, preferably in a supervised facility like a hotel.

---

[22] https://www.chronicle.com/article/Here-s-a-List-of-Colleges-/248626

Have any countries had success in reopening safely? What led to their success?

The countries leading the way in reopening their cities are, for the most part, those that were able to quickly contain the disease when it first began to spread.

In Taiwan, China, and South Korea, a combination of government-supported public health measures, smart technologies, and consistent engagement with the general public has paved the way for current attempts to resume social and economic activity. While only time will tell whether their respective reopening can be judged a true "success," the number of new cases reported daily continues to drop in all three countries.[cxvi]

One component that is largely present in these successful disease control efforts are designated isolation centers where people who have been infected or exposed can quarantine.[cxvii] Two other vital components, testing and contact tracing, are present in the U.S. response but not nearly as widespread or robust.

What happens if a country reopens before the epidemic has subsided?

If rates of infection are still high, it is very likely that they will increase. Within weeks, the number of confirmed cases and hospitalizations will surge, as will death rates.

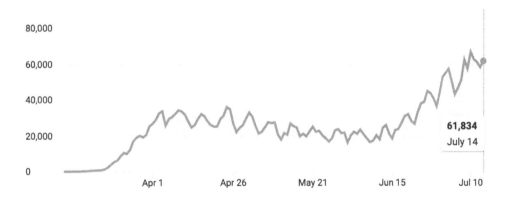

Telemedicine

What is telehealth or telemedicine?

Telehealth or telemedicine takes processes that constitute healthcare as we know it—visits to the clinic, exchanges of health information, health education—and conducts them remotely, using telecommunications technology. It includes a consultation completed over phone or video chat as much as a mobile health application that allows you to access your health data online.

Telemedicine can be used to reach patients in remote locations and reduce congestion at clinics and other healthcare facilities. Usually, telemedicine is a format most suited to follow-up visits, medication, chronic disease management, and other kinds of consultations that can be conducted virtually.

In most cases, a respiratory syndrome like Covid can be evaluated and detected using telemedicine.

How common is telemedicine?

Thanks to Covid, about half of physicians across the country are now using telemedicine to continue caring for their patients.[cxviii] Not all providers have the technological or administrative capabilities to make a transition so abrupt, but many are having to find a solution fast—or risk losing contact or continuity of care. Visits to clinics and other outpatient care centers have plummeted since the beginning of March, putting some practices in dire straits.[cxix]

Many U.S. insurers have expanded their policies to cover more telehealth services in the wake of the pandemic. For example, Blue Cross Blue Shield of Massachusetts, a private health insurance company, expanded its policy to include more coverage for telemedicine in March. As of May 21, Blue Cross has processed upwards of a million telehealth claims, which amount to tens of thousands per day.[cxx]

To see how different insurance providers are taking action around Covid, check out the guide created by America's Health Insurance Plans that is linked at the bottom of the page.[23]

More health systems are expected to adopt some form of telemedicine both during and after the pandemic, with the number of telehealth visits predicted to increase more than five times over for 2020.[cxxi]

How can telemedicine help during Covid? What are its limitations?

One benefit is that people who suspect they might have Covid but aren't sure can consult with their doctor without

---

[23] https://www.ahip.org/health-insurance-providers-respond-to-coronavirus-covid-19/

risking unnecessary exposure in a waiting or examination room.

But telemedicine, like traditional health services, is not readily available or accessible to everyone—even though it tends to be marketed as a tool for closing the gaps that fragment our systems of care.

The digital divide that exists between those who have a stable internet connection and those who don't is one barrier. Others include a lack of functioning electronics and basic technological literacy. These are especially rife in rural and low-income communities, whose residents generally suffer from some of the greatest health disparities in the country.

Working and Learning from Home

How can I create an ideal environment for working from home?

To start, focus on your immediate environment. Make a habit of decluttering your desk space or desktop before you get down to business or do some simple list-making to get your priorities straight. Remember—your mind needs just as much upkeep as your surroundings.

Experts recommend devoting a few minutes each day to a gratitude, mindfulness, or meditation practice, or a combination of those, to mentally reset before or after a long workday. For more tips on working from home, check out the guide created by Healthline.[24]

What are some easy ways I can give my brain a break?

Try breaking your schedule up into uninterrupted chunks of work time punctuated by short breaks. One variation of this is the famous Pomodoro Technique, in which every 25 to 30

---

[24] https://www.healthline.com/health/working-from-home-tips#tips-for-newbies

minutes of work time is met with a five-minute pause.[cxxii] Some people prefer longer chunks of an hour or two. The key is to stop and rest at consistent intervals, whether that means drinking water, grabbing a snack, or having a quick stretch.

How can I avoid burnout while working from home?

When it comes to introducing some breathing room into an overwhelming work schedule, it can be the little things that count. If a commute to and from your place of work once served that purpose, try slotting in some open-ended "commute time" that will help you ease in and out of work mode. Allow yourself time to recharge on the weekends. If the weather is nice and you have a spare minute, go for a walk with a mask or face shield and at a safe distance from others to unwind.

Ultimately, the trick is to find an approach that works for you and stick with it. To get a sense of how widely such strategies can vary, check out the website listed at the bottom of the page that was compiled using the advice of business leaders and wellbeing experts across the country.[25]

How do I balance working from home with helping my kids with their remote learning?

At the beginning of each day and week, compare your work schedule with your kid's learning schedule and, as best you can, set your priorities and plan time accordingly. Kids benefit from routine—as will you—so being able to create and fall into a consistent rhythm is your best bet at introducing some structure into your new situation, inevitable interruptions aside.

---

[25] https://thriveglobal.com/stories/how-to-avoid-burnout-stress-work-from-home-tips/

When it works, square your kids away with learning and extracurricular activities to keep them busy so you can have long periods of uninterrupted focus. Some days will demand more intervention on your part than others, making it extremely difficult to be productive—and that's okay.

For more tips on how to juggle work and your kid's education from experts and parents alike, check out the guide compiled by *Vox*.[26]

What if my kid doesn't enjoy virtual learning and virtual playdates?

Chances are your kid isn't allergic to the technology itself, but instead tired of not being able to go to school and play with friends like they did before. If their sadness or frustration is beginning to affect their ability to participate in

---

[26] https://www.vox.com/identities/2020/3/25/21193142/coronavirus-covid-19-kids-work-from-home-child-care-school-cancellations

school and have fun, there are a few things you can try out that might help.

Remember that even if you've had conversations with your child about the pandemic and its impact on our social and emotional lives, they still might lack the language they need to process these changes and express their feelings about them. Helping them find that language might not cure their aversion to Zoom, but it would at least help you both understand it.

For more advice from experts on how to respond to your kid's aversion to virtual hangouts, check out *HuffPost's* guide.[27]

---

[27] https://www.huffpost.com/entry/zoom-and-google-hangouts-are-making-kids-miserable_l_5ebd5cbbc5b655620b13a149?utm_campaign=share_email&ncid=other_email_o63gt2jcad4

Summer Safety

Across the Northern Hemisphere, temperatures are on the rise, and in some parts of the world, Covid cases are on the decline. Where the pandemic has receded, lockdowns have lifted—and for those lucky enough to live there, the slow, unsteady process of "going back to normal" begins.

Normally, summertime gives us an excuse to let loose: to wear less, go out more, and take time off for a vacation long overdue. While ebbs in the past months' restrictions offer some form of relief, health authorities local and global have made one thing clear. This battle is far from over; weary as we are, vigilance is needed to keep the enemy at bay.

Humans are nothing if not resourceful, and where there is a will to make summer fun, there is always a way. In this case, blind resolve and tunnel vision will get us nowhere. What can and will carry us forward is our ability to step back and look around—to survey our surroundings, spot signs of danger, and know when to advance and when to retreat.

"Personal risk" is public health's new catchphrase, and so long as we learn how to gauge it, this summer can be as active and adventurous as any other. In name, personal risk centers the individual. But in practice, it requires awareness of—and compassion for—everyone but. That could be a spouse or coworker; a schoolteacher or janitor; a neighboring city or far-off country.

There are ways to let loose and enjoy a bit of life that don't risk anyone else's. What follows is a guide that can show you how.

Questions Kids Ask Us

Are things going back to normal now?

In many parts of the world, the disease is dying down. People living in these places are starting to go out again and do fun things. As long as they keep doing what they need to do to protect themselves and the people around them, the disease will leave them alone.

But in other parts of the world, more people are getting the disease than before. And there are even some countries, like the United States, where both things are happening at once. Some states are getting better, while others are getting worse.

This is why you need to keep wearing a mask, social distancing, and washing your hands a lot, even if you live in a place where you're allowed to spend more and more time outdoors. That way, everyone stays safe.

It's so hot outside. Do I have to wear my mask all the time?

You do most of the time. Whenever other people are around, you need to keep your mask on, no matter how hot it is.

Can I wear a face shield instead?

Yes. Face shields are easier to wear than masks when it's hot out. They protect your eyes better than masks do, and everything else just as well.

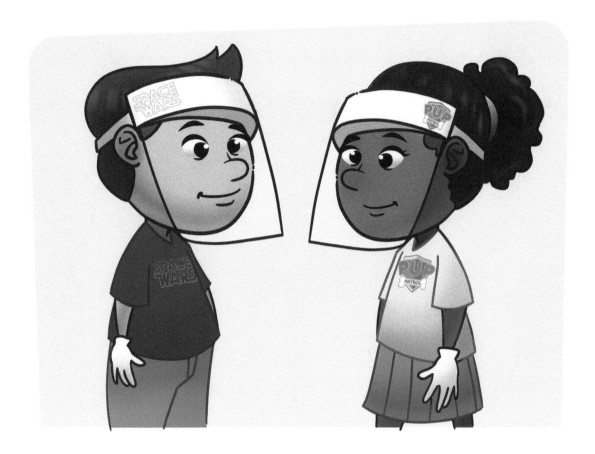

When am I allowed to take my mask or face shield off outside?

It is better to keep them on. But if no one else is around, you can.

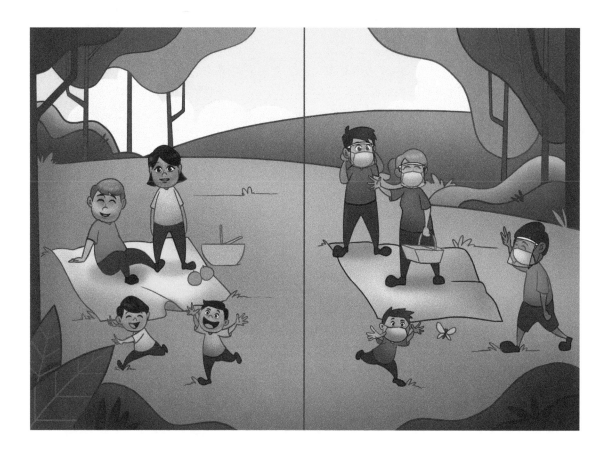

Can I go to the playground?

Yes, as long as you're with your parents and the playground isn't too crowded. The playground should also be close to your house.

If only a few kids are around, stay six feet away from anyone who isn't family. Use hand sanitizer often and keep your mask on at all times.

Can I play sports?

On your own and with other people in your household, yes. But team sports you play at school or with friends, like basketball and soccer, won't be safe to play for a while.

Sports you can play without getting close to anyone else, like tennis, are safe as long as you don't share equipment and play outside.

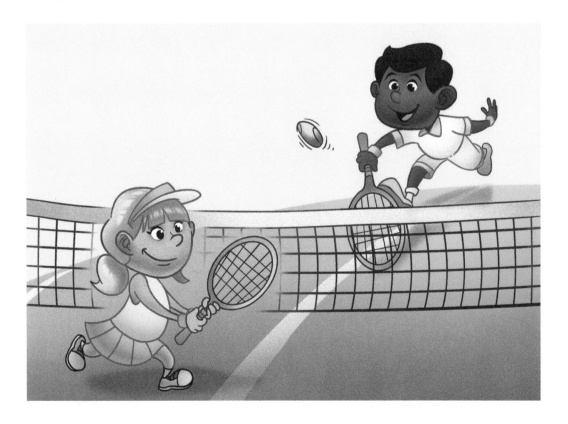

If I'm swimming, do I have to wear my mask in the water?

No. It gets hard to breathe if your mask is wet, which is dangerous. That's why you should bring two masks whenever you go swimming, just in case.

Whenever you're in the water, wear your usual goggles and swim masks instead.

Can I go to the beach or a lake?

Yes, as long as your parents think the water is clean and you and your family keep at least six feet of distance from other people.

If other people are around, remember to wear a mask when you're not in the water.

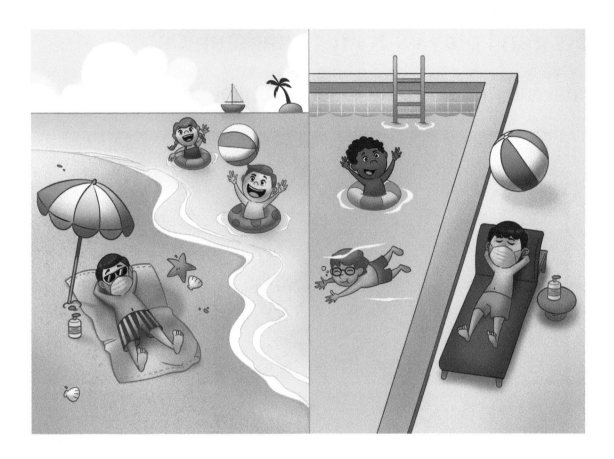

Can I go to the pool?

You have to be very careful when going swimming in a public pool. The water may not be clean and there may be many people there.

Can I still go to summer camp?

This summer, it probably isn't safe.

How can I play with my friends and stay safe?

Find a fun game to play together online instead!

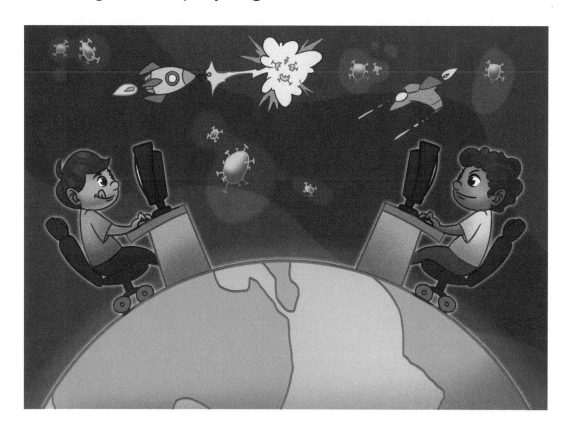

Questions We Ask Ourselves

SITUATIONAL AWARENESS

The information below is directly reprinted from Part Two.

Covid is still a global threat. Until the day that this is no longer the case, we all have a responsibility to stay informed about the dangers this disease presents to our communities, our loved ones, and ourselves. Following certain rules isn't enough to guarantee our safety. We must understand why the rules are there to begin with, and how they change depending on where we are, who we are, and what we're doing.

The first thing we must learn is *situational awareness*. What is the rate of infection in your community, and how likely is it that you're going to encounter someone who is infected?

Start by finding the daily number of new Covid cases in your area at the smallest scale possible—whether it's your county, or your zip code. Using this data, calculate the average number of new cases for the past week. Multiply that number by 10, and you'll have a rough idea of how many people in your community are currently infected.

If the average daily number of new cases is very low—somewhere in the range of 10 to 20—then you can consider yourself relatively safe and free to resume your daily activities. Even though you should continue taking appropriate precautions, you no longer need to isolate at home. If the average daily number of new cases is 50 to 100, you'll need to be more careful. Any number higher than that, and you'll need to be *much* more careful.

In addition to building situational awareness, we must learn to gauge our *personal risk*. Do you have any underlying health conditions that put you at risk? Then you'll need to stay at home as much as possible. A related factor is the *risk of people around you*. Does anyone you're living with have underlying health conditions that put them at risk? If so, your actions will impact them directly.

Whenever you enter a new setting—whether it's your place of work or your child's school—these same factors must be reevaluated, and the risk recalculated. Consider the coworkers on your floor, or the classmates, teachers, janitors, and bus drivers who shuffle in, out, and around the school your child attends. Where are they coming from? What is their risk? If they're at risk, so are you.

Last but not least, we must learn and think critically about the precautions being taken in these settings to keep us safe. Take your child's school. What are they doing to prevent infection, and what will do in the event that infection occurs? Are they conducting temperature screenings? Insisting that students and staff wear masks or face shields? What about social distancing? Don't be afraid to ask questions and, if you're dissatisfied with the answers, advocate for a better solution.

The complex *hierarchy of risk* I describe above can be broken down into the questions below:

1. **How many people are infected on a daily basis in my community?** Remember, multiply by 10 to get a rough estimate of the number of active infections.

2. **Am I or someone in my household at higher risk?**

3. **Will the activity be indoors or outdoors?** The risk is 20 times higher indoors than outdoors.

4. **How long will I be there?** The shorter, the better—especially if the activity is indoors.

5. **How many people will be there?** The fewer, the better.

6. **Will they be wearing masks or face shields?** For an activity to be safe, especially if it's indoors, the answer must be yes.

7. **What precautions are staff, hosts, administrators, or whoever is in charge taking to ensure my safety?**

EVALUATING RISK

How do I figure out I my personal risk level?

At any moment, your personal risk level depends on several factors (see the checklist above). These include your age and medical history, as well as where you live, who you live with, what you're doing, where you're doing it—just to name a few.

Some organizations have created handy infographics that help us gauge the risk level of different activities more easily. On the following page is one made by the Texas Medical Association.

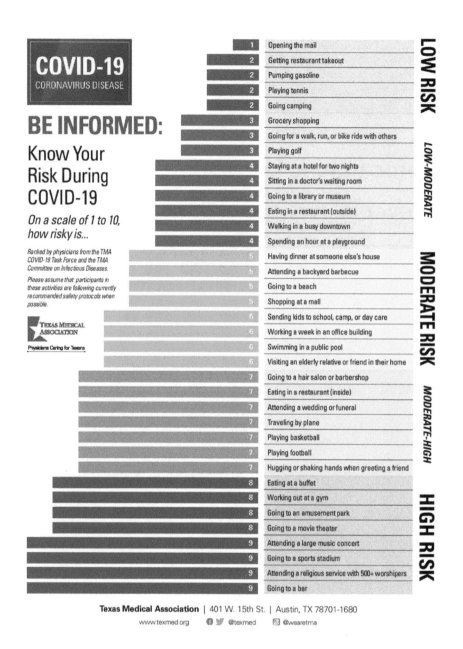

Source: Texas Medical Association, July 2020, https://www.texmed.org/coronavirus/

Is it safer to be outside than inside?

That depends on where you are. If you live in an area where case counts are still high or on the rise, it's in your best interest to stay at home as much as possible.

But if you live in an area where rates of infection have dropped significantly, businesses have reopened successfully, and people are beginning to socialize and gather together again, many outdoor activities will not only be safe, but *much safer than indoor alternatives*. The key is to continue following the safety guidelines put out by local health authorities, which generally involve wearing masks and social distancing but vary from activity to activity.

The risk involved with many kinds of summer fun doesn't so much concern the great outdoors as it does the indoor facilities that accompany them. For example: going to the beach is risky not because the Covid virus can brave the heat, but because beachgoers tend to overcrowd nearby restaurants and bars after they've had their fill of sand and surf.

Why is it so much safer to socialize outside than inside?

Indoors, the virus-laden droplets you and anyone else expels tend to hang around in the air. Outdoors, the same droplets can be scattered and killed by sun and wind.

One report estimates the chances of catching the virus to be *20 times greater indoors than outdoors*—a statistic too startling to ignore.[cxxiii] That finding echoes those of several other studies that traced clusters and outbreaks of Covid cases back to mostly indoor environments.[cxxiv]

When do I need to wear a mask or face shield?

If you're going to be near people outside your household—even if you're six feet apart—you should keep your mask on at all times.

Only if no one is around, or if you're only with people who belong to your household, is it then safe to take off your mask.

You should also remove your mask when you're swimming, though you must remember to put it back on once you're out of the water.[cxxv]

Is it safe to eat at restaurants now?

Ordering food to go is still safer than dining in.

If you do want to dine in, choose a restaurant where you can eat outside.[cxxvi] Many restaurants that didn't offer outdoor seating prior to the pandemic are now doing so. But regardless of whether you're eating inside or outside, you need to make sure your table is at least six feet from the next.

As soon as you get to the restaurant, wash your hands. Wash them before you leave, too. While dining, keep your mask on as much as possible, especially if you're inside.

Can I still pick up some summer reading from my local library?

As much as you can, take advantage of any curbside pickup services or digital materials, like eBooks and audiobooks, that your library has to offer.[cxxvii] The same goes for online catalogs that allow you to browse and reserve items from the safety of your phone or computer.

Can I use computers or laptops at my local library?

This isn't recommended. But if you do use a public computer station, the U.S. Centers for Disease Control and Prevention recommends using disinfectant wipes to swipe stray germs of the mouse and keyboard first.[cxxviii]

What are some places and activities I should avoid?

Don't go anywhere or attend anything that tends to draw a huge crowd, like a large music concert or sports stadium.

Also avoid indoor venues like movie theatres and gyms.

OUTDOOR ACTIVITIES

Which outdoor activities are broadly considered safe?

If you keep your distance from others, exercising outside is safe. Bike riding, jogging, or hiking are all safe activities as long as you keep your distance. You must always be very wary of shared bathrooms.

If you want to play sports, stick to the ones that permit six feet of distance from other players. Use your own equipment and don't share it with others. Sanitize your hands regularly, and don't forget to disinfect your equipment before and after each game.

What is the safest way to host an outdoor gathering?

We know by now that being outdoors isn't enough. Long before the summer began and certainly ever since, new clusters of Covid cases have been linked to midsize gatherings of family and friends—even when the party was taken outside.[cxxix]

To stay safe, keep the number of attendees low. Have everyone, yourself included, wear a mask at all times. Don't share utensils or even food; ask your guests to bring their own.

The New York Times has published a guide to hosting a socially distanced barbecue that is linked at the bottom of the page.[28]

Can I go to the gym?

This is one activity I would not recommend. As long as the pandemic prevails, exercising at home or outside around the neighborhood will be safer than going to the gym.

If you must go to the gym, call before you visit to ask about the precautions they're taking to prevent infection. If they've set up an online system for reservations and check-ins, use it—and if outdoor facilities are available, use them.

Whether you're working out inside or outside, stay six feet away from everyone else and disinfect any equipment before you use it. Wear a mask when you can.[cxxx]

---

[28] https://www.nytimes.com/2020/06/26/dining/social-distance-bbq-recipes.html?smid=em-share

What if I'm not used to exercising outside when it's hot?

Exercising outside may be more uncomfortable, but it is also a good deal safer. And if you schedule your workout for the early morning or evening, you might even beat the heat.

Just remember to stay hydrated and, whenever you need to, take it down a notch and go slow. Your body will adjust, but it might take time.[cxxxi]

What about outdoor activities that involve food, like farmers markets?

Farmers markets are safe as long as both visitors and vendors wear masks and stay six feet apart.

Fresh produce is very unlikely to transmit the virus, but its handlers should still use gloves. If you're a customer, don't touch produce or other products unless you're purchasing them, and don't forget to wash or sanitize your purchases once you get home.

Is it safe to bring my kids to a playground?

The latest guidelines from the U.S. Centers for Disease Control and Prevention tell us that the safety of playgrounds is difficult to guarantee—especially when they're crawling with kids.[cxxxii] Rules on the specifics of use and disinfection vary from state to state.[cxxxiii]

If you do choose to bring your kids to a playground, visit once close to home when it's not crowded and bring plenty of hand sanitizer. As long as you keep a close eye on your children and everyone keeps their masks on, the risk of infection should remain low.

Can young kids start to have playdates again?

What makes playdates trickier—and perhaps riskier—than other social activities is how unpredictable young kids can be. Even if you communicate thoroughly with your kids, other parents, and their kids about rules and expectations, there can be no guarantee that all will go as planned.

The first step to planning a playdate is having an honest conversation with any other parents or caregivers about safety and risk. Just because infection rates in your community are low doesn't mean everyone is prepared to accept a new level of exposure.

If it is clear that all parties are willing, lay down some ground rules: no sharing, no touching, lots of hand sanitizing, six feet of distance, masks on always, and so on. Outside is better than inside, and adult supervision is a must. Again, no matter how meticulously you plan, safety won't be guaranteed.[cxxxiv]

What about teenagers who want to hang out with their friends?

I wouldn't recommend it. Teens can be impulsive. Left to their own devices, they might make poor choices.

What about public swimming pools?

One of the many ways this virus can spread is through the *oral fecal route.*[cxxxv] This occurs when virus from the feces of one person infects another person by mouth, usually by means of contaminated water.

The problem with public pools is that many people are swimming around in the same, small body of water—and unfortunately, that water isn't difficult to contaminate. All it takes is one kid who doesn't wipe properly.

Ideally, local health officials and pool staff will work together to follow the guidelines published by the U.S. Centers for Disease Control and Prevention and keep pools disinfected and safe.[cxxxvi] But since compliance isn't guaranteed, take care to avoid crowds.

If I do go to a swimming pool, how can I keep myself and my children safe?

Stay six feet away from strangers, wear your mask whenever you're not in the water, and steer clear of damp, enclosed spaces like locker rooms and showers. If you're bringing children, keep an even closer eye on them than usual.

Is it safe to go swimming in a lake or ocean?

In general, yes. But to know whether a specific lake or ocean is safe to swim in, you'll need to check its *coliform count*.

Rainstorms can usher overflows of raw sewage into lakes and oceans. That's why each day, environmental health authorities must measure their *E. coli levels*, or their coliform count. Coliform bacteria, otherwise known as E. coli, is found in human feces, which makes it a good indicator of contamination.

Before taking a dip in a nearby lake or ocean, call your environmental health authorities and ask about the E. coli levels reported that day. If you live in the United States, a state-by-state list of health and environmental agencies is linked at the bottom of the page.[29]

Is it safe to go to the beach?

Yes, but you must take certain precautions to keep your risk level as low as possible.

If you live in the United States, visit the website of the U.S. Environmental Protection Agency to find the safest beaches

---

[29] https://www.epa.gov/home/health-and-environmental-agencies-us-states-and-territories

in your area.[30] Their website is a gateway to information on water quality, closures, and health advisories that will be crucial for planning a safe beach trip.

When picking which beach to visit, make social distancing a priority. If a beach is known to draw crowds, best to avoid it and opt for one where a minimum of six feet of distance from staff and other visitors is guaranteed. Do not, under any circumstances, share food, toys, sunscreen, or other materials with anyone other than the people you live with.[cxxxvii]

Once at the beach, you'll want to keep your mask on if you're not in the water and people outside your household are around. But if you manage to find an isolated spot, no mask is needed.

---

[30] https://www.epa.gov/beaches/find-information-about-particular-us-beach

When you're fixing to leave, resist the impulse to head to the nearest restaurant or bar after being in the sun all day. Bars especially are breeding grounds for infection. Retire instead to your home.

Is it safe for my kids to go to summer camp?

The ideal summer camp would be very small, with all campers coming from a nearby area. Campers would have to stay six feet apart at all times and engage mostly in outdoor activities.[cxxxviii]

If your go-to summer camp fails to meet these requirements, it might be a good idea to hold off enrolling this year.

Is it safe to have a picnic?

Absolutely—as long as you're (a) with the people in your household, and (b) parking your picnic blanket six feet away from others or, better yet, in a secluded area.

Having picnics with people outside your household, however, is not recommended. If you do have a picnic, all parties must bring their own food, stay six feet apart, and keep their masks on unless they're eating. For more advice, check out *The New York Times*' guide on the topic.[31]

What about a barbecue?

Because barbecuing is such a popular—and, during the pandemic at least, risky—summer activity, even the U.S. Centers for Disease Control and Prevention has released guidelines on how to host a safe barbecue.

In summary, they advise us to tell sick or recently recovered invitees to stay at home; organize seating and direct traffic so all guests are constantly six feet apart; wear masks when not eating; set up and clearly mark designated hand

---

[31] https://www.nytimes.com/2020/05/09/dining/coronavirus-how-to-have-a-picnic-safely.html

sanitizing and handwashing stations; and limit opportunities for sharing and handling food.

The additional guidelines—on how to eliminate high-touch surfaces, for example—are worth reading and available on the U.S. Centers for Disease Control and Prevention website.[32]

Is it safe to go hiking?

Done right, a socially distanced hike can not only be great exercise, but very safe. While most national parks and other natural wonders that tend to draw crowds will probably stay closed for the summer, there remains a great opportunity to explore nearby trails and parks you might overlook otherwise.

---

[32] https://www.cdc.gov/coronavirus/2019-ncov/daily-life-coping/personal-social-activities.html

For extensive and easy-to-understand advice on how to plan a safe solo or family hike, check out the American Hiking Society's guide, "Hiking and Playing Outside in the Time of COVID-19".[33]

Is it safe to go fishing or boating?

If you go alone or with members of your household, yes. Restrictions may apply depending on where you live, however.

Is it safe to go camping?

Some states are beginning to open up their camp sites, though this is happening on a case-by-case basis. It will take a lot of planning to make your camping trip safe, but as long as you're careful, it will be preferable to staying at a hotel or vacationing in an urban area.

---

[33] https://americanhiking.org/blog/hiking-responsibly-faq-covid-19/

To get a better idea of what you, and operators of campgrounds, need to do to camp safely, consult out the guidelines compiled by the Minnesota Department of Natural Resources linked at the bottom of the page.[34]

TRAVEL

Is it safe to go on a vacation?

Consider the following factors:

Where you are and where you're going: Neither your current place of residence nor your destination should have a high rate of infection. Avoid cities and other densely populated areas. To play it safest, go camping.

How you're getting there: If you want to travel safely, take a car. Avoid flying and public transport.

---

[34] https://staysafe.mn.gov/assets/campgrounds-guidance_tcm1152-435378.pdf

Where you stay: Avoid hotels if you can.

What is the safest way to travel?

As of now, the safest way to travel is in your own car.

Is it safe to go on a road trip with friends or another family?

If you want to go on a road trip with someone outside of your household, use different cars, as you will be sitting in a confined space for several hours.

Don't get into a car with anyone you haven't been sequestered with

If I'm traveling a great distance by car, which public restrooms are safe for me to use?

While some places are taking precautions like setting up portable toilets, roping off some sinks, or sanitizing their restrooms every half hour, there isn't a way to ensure that a public restroom remains virus-free.[cxxxix]

If you do need to use a public restroom, keep your mask on, use a paper towel when touching any surfaces, and of course give your hands a good wash on your way out.

If I'm driving a long distance, is it safe to stay at hotels or rental properties along the way?

Staying overnight in a hotel or rented apartment is risky. You can never be sure of who was there before you and how well the space was cleaned. Until the number of new infections at all points of your destination is very low— between zero to five per day—I would not recommend traveling unless it is absolutely necessary.

If you do need to stay at a hotel, call in advance and ask about the protective measures they're taking to keep guests safe. Once you arrive, stay away from common areas like the hotel lobby and avoid interacting with anyone outside your party.

If I'm traveling by plane, how do I keep myself safe?

It is very difficult to guarantee your safety on a plane. At least for now, there is no guarantee as to how you will be seated and how clean the plane will be.

If you must travel by plane, keep your mask on at all times as long as you're in the airport. To be even safer, wear tight-fitting goggles and a face shield.

When you go through a security checkpoint, a TSA official on duty may ask you to lower your mask or remove your protective gear. But otherwise, keep it on. Shopping or eating at airport restaurants isn't advised. Bring your own food, books, and eye drops instead.

Once on the plane, keep your mask on as much as possible. Wipe your seat down with disinfecting wipes before you sit in it.

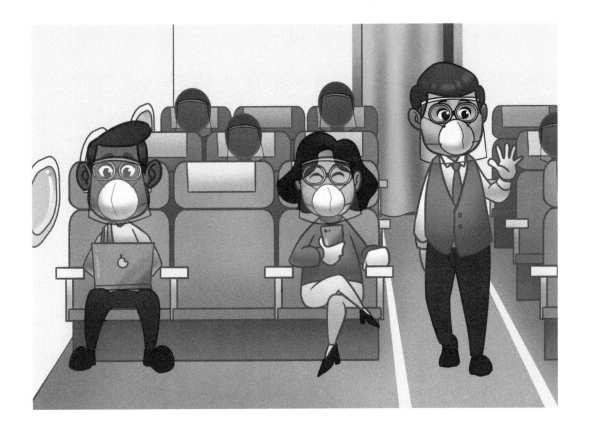

Are people who live in the United States banned from traveling to Europe?

As of this writing, yes. For visitors from countries like Japan and Canada, the European Union has reopened its borders as of July 1. But for Americans, they remain closed due to soaring case counts.[cxl] Only a select few groups, including health professionals, diplomats, and those who hold long-term visas, are exempt.[cxli]

Because the United Kingdom exited the European Union in January, the ban doesn't extend there. There is currently no word on when the ban will end.

PART THREE

Resources

KIDS

Covid-19 Education

Dr. Panda TotoTime

https://www.youtube.com/channel/UCpzdzxPD8acq8ssStKvDNtw

BrainPOP – Coronavirus

https://www.brainpop.com/health/diseasesinjuriesandconditions/coronavirus/

PBS for Parents – Science

https://www.pbs.org/parents/learn-grow/all-ages/science

ADULTS

Covid Information Hubs

U.S. Centers for Disease Control:

https://www.cdc.gov/coronavirus/2019-ncov/index.html

U.S. Food and Drug Administration:

https://www.fda.gov/emergency-preparedness-and-response/counterterrorism-and-emerging-threats/coronavirus-disease-2019-covid-19

World Health Organization:

https://www.who.int/emergencies/diseases/novel-coronavirus-2019

National Coalition of STD Directors: Maps, graphs, and figures about coronavirus. https://www.ncsddc.org/covid-command-center-maps-graphs-figures/

Interactive Maps and Lists

See How All 50 States Are Reopening

https://www.nytimes.com/interactive/2020/us/states-reopen-map-coronavirus.html

Here's a List of Colleges' Plans for Reopening in the Fall

https://www.chronicle.com/article/Here-s-a-List-of-Colleges-/248626

Health Insurance Providers Respond to Coronavirus (COVID-19) https://www.ahip.org/health-insurance-providers-respond-to-coronavirus-covid-19/

Disinfectants for Use Against SARS-CoV-2 (COVID-19)

https://www.epa.gov/pesticide-registration/list-n-disinfectants-use-against-sars-cov-2-covid-19

Personal Protective Equipment EUAs

https://www.fda.gov/medical-devices/coronavirus-disease-2019-covid-19-emergency-use-authorizations-medical-devices/personal-protective-equipment-euas

Fraudulent Coronavirus Disease 2019 (COVID-19) Products https://www.fda.gov/consumers/health-fraud-scams/fraudulent-coronavirus-disease-2019-covid-19-products

Coronavirus Shutdown https://www.coronashutdown.com/

Covid ActNow https://covidactnow.org/?s=37528

Staying Safe

Worker Safety and Support

https://www.cdc.gov/coronavirus/2019-ncov/community/worker-safety-support/index.html

Disinfectants for Use Against SARS-CoV-2 (COVID-19)

https://www.epa.gov/pesticide-registration/list-n-disinfectants-use-against-sars-cov-2-covid-19

How to Make Cloth Face Coverings

https://www.cdc.gov/coronavirus/2019-ncov/prevent-getting-sick/how-to-make-cloth-face-covering.html

How Often You Should Wash Your Sheets During The Coronavirus Pandemic

https://www.huffpost.com/entry/how-often-wash-sheets-coronavirus-pandemic_l_5eac4f6bc5b624b396929d10?utm_campaign=share_email&ncid=other_email_o63gt2jcad4

What We Know About Face Shields and Coronavirus

https://www.wsj.com/articles/what-we-know-about-face-shields-and-coronavirus-11592321931?st=i4dcpazmkmnudz0&reflink=article_email_share

A User's Guide to Face Masks

https://www.nytimes.com/2020/04/10/well/live/coronavirus-face-masks-guides-protection-personal-protective-equipment.html?smid=em-share

Specific Health Conditions

Coronavirus (COVID-19) and People with HIV

https://www.hiv.gov/hiv-basics/staying-in-hiv-care/other-related-health-issues/coronavirus-covid-19

COVID-19 and HIV https://www.cdc.gov/hiv/covid-19/index.html

If You Are Immunocompromised, Protect Yourself From COVID-19 https://www.cdc.gov/coronavirus/2019-ncov/need-extra-precautions/immunocompromised.html

COVID-19 Guidance for People Who Use Drugs and Harm Reduction Programs

https://harmreduction.org/miscellaneous/covid-19-guidance-for-people-who-use-drugs-and-harm-reduction-programs/

Parenting

Kids Are Grieving, Too

https://www.nytimes.com/2020/05/13/parenting/kids-death-coronavirus-grieving.html?smid=em-share

When coronavirus strikes, kids make the news

https://www.washingtonpost.com/graphics/2020/lifestyle/kidspost/kids-newspapers-coronavirus/

A Kids' Guide to Coronavirus (podcast episode)

https://www.nytimes.com/2020/03/27/podcasts/the-daily/kids-coronavirus.html?searchResultPosition=1

Kids Are So Over Zoom. Here's What To Do About It.

https://www.huffpost.com/entry/zoom-and-google-hangouts-are-making-kids-miserable_l_5ebd5cbbc5b655620b13a149?utm_campaign=share_email&ncid=other_email_o63gt2jcad4

6 Tips You Can Trust: How to help kids cope with extended school closures

https://www.savethechildren.org/content/dam/usa/reports/e

mergency-response/help-kids-cope-with-school-closures.pdf

Pets

Pet Safety & COVID-19

https://www.youtube.com/watch?v=KHMYC5Comio&feature=emb_logo

Pregnancy and Infant Care

When Can Grandparents Meet the Newborn?

https://www.nytimes.com/2020/06/16/parenting/baby/grandparents-meet-newborn-coronavirus.html

Navigating Your Pregnancy: Coping with stress and anxiety during the Covid-19 pandemic

https://www.marchofdimes.org/it-starts-with-mom/coping-with-stress-and-anxiety-during-the-covid-19-pandemic.aspx

Covid-19 Psychological Wellness Guide: Pregnant Mothers

https://med.emory.edu/departments/psychiatry/_documents/tips.pregnant.mothers.pdf

Maternal Mental Health Leadership Alliance Covid-19 Resource Directory https://www.mmhla.org/covid-19/

Mental Health

COVID-19 Resource and Information Guide

https://www.nami.org/Support-Education/NAMI-HelpLine/COVID-19-Information-and-Resources/COVID-19-Resource-and-Information-Guide

Distant Together: Mental Health Resources for COVID-19

https://www.distanttogether.org/

Why Uncertainty Feels So Terrifying, And How To Cope With It https://www.huffpost.com/entry/uncertainty-stress-how-to-cope_l_5ed0047cc5b6521c93a80e43?utm_campaign=share_email&ncid=other_email_o63gt2jcad4

How To Sleep Better If Coronavirus Anxiety Is Keeping You Awake https://www.huffpost.com/entry/sleep-better-coronavirus-anxiety_l_5e8b5b2cc5b6cc1e47799a4d

Dealing With Coronavirus Anxiety? Here Are Some Ways To Cope With The Stress

https://www.huffpost.com/entry/coronavirus-anxiety-stress-tips_l_5e84a845c5b6a1bb76512b7d

What Not To Say To Someone Grieving During The Coronavirus Crisis https://www.huffpost.com/entry/what-not-to-say-grieving-coronavirus_l_5ea9a134c5b6fb98a2b65056?utm_campaign=share_email&ncid=other_email_o63gt2jcad4

10 Sneaky Ways Your Coronavirus Anxiety Is Coming Out https://www.huffingtonpost.co.uk/entry/10-sneaky-ways-your-coronavirus-anxiety-is-coming-

out_uk_5ec50185c5b6c1f21e70dd93?utm_campaign=shar e_email&ncid=other_email_o63gt2jcad4&guccounter=1

Why Uncertainty Feels So Terrifying, And How To Cope With It https://www.huffpost.com/entry/uncertainty-stress-how-to-cope_l_5ed0047cc5b6521c93a80e43?utm_campaign=sha re_email&ncid=other_email_o63gt2jcad4

Working from Home

26 WFH Tips While Self-Isolating During the COVID-19 Outbreak https://www.healthline.com/health/working-from-home-tips#tips-for-newbies

Working from home with kids feels unsustainable. Here's how to ease the burden. https://www.vox.com/identities/2020/3/25/21193142/coron avirus-covid-19-kids-work-from-home-child-care-school-cancellations

How to Set Boundaries and Avoid Burnout While Working From Home https://thriveglobal.com/stories/how-to-avoid-burnout-stress-work-from-home-tips/

Helping Others

Ways to help older neighbors and relatives in isolation (and how they can help you) https://www.washingtonpost.com/lifestyle/2020/05/06/seniors-isolation-quarantine-help-how-to/

BIBLIOGRAPHY

Summer Section

Caron, Christina. "As Playgrounds Start to Reopen, Here's How to Keep Kids Safe." *New York Times*, June 11, 2020. Accessed July 14, 2020. https://www.nytimes.com/2020/06/11/parenting/playgrounds-reopen-safety-coronavirus.html?smid=em-share.

Elliott, Christopher. "Everything Americans need to know about the E.U. travel ban." *Washington Post*, July 8, 2020. Accessed July 14, 2020. https://www.washingtonpost.com/lifestyle/travel/everything-americans-need-to-know-about-the-eu-travel-ban/2020/07/08/8fea554e-bc89-11ea-80b9-40ece9a701dc_story.html.

European Commission. "Travel to and from the EU during the pandemic." European Commission website. Last modified June 2020. Accessed July 14, 2020. https://ec.europa.eu/info/live-work-travel-eu/health/coronavirus-response/travel-and-transportation-during-coronavirus-pandemic/travel-and-eu-during-pandemic_en#exemption-details.

Harvard Medical School. "Coronavirus outbreak and kids." Harvard Health Publishing. Last modified July 2, 2020. Accessed July 14, 2020.

https://www.health.harvard.edu/diseases-and-conditions/coronavirus-outbreak-and-kids.

Nishiura, Hiroshi, Hitoshi Oshitani, Tetsuro Kobayashi, Tomoya Saito, Tomimasa Sunagawa, Tamano Matsui, Takaji Wakita, MHLW COVID-19 Response Team, and Motoi Suzuki. "Closed environments facilitate secondary transmission of coronavirus disease 2019 (COVID-19)." *medRxiv*, April 16, 2020. Accessed July 14, 2020. https://doi.org/10.1101/2020.02.28.20029272.

Parker-Pope, Tara. "How Safe Are Outdoor Gatherings?" *New York Times*, July 3, 2020. Accessed July 14, 2020. https://www.nytimes.com/2020/07/03/well/live/coronavirus-spread-outdoors-party.html?smid=em-share.

Potkewitz, Hilary. "How to Exercise Safely Outdoors in the Heat." *Wall Street Journal*, July 12, 2020. Accessed July 14, 2020. https://www.wsj.com/articles/how-to-exercise-safely-outdoors-in-the-heat-11594551600?st=juvahmsij2hrnci&reflink=article_email_share.

Qian, Hua, Te Miao, Li Liu, Xiaohong Zheng, Danting Luo, and Yuguo Li. "Indoor transmission of SARS-CoV-2." *medRxiv*, April 7, 2020. Accessed July 14, 2020. https://doi.org/10.1101/2020.04.04.20053058.

Teitell, Beth. "We can take road trips now. But where are we supposed to go to the bathroom?" *Boston Globe*, June 8, 2020. Accessed July 14, 2020.

https://www.bostonglobe.com/2020/06/08/nation/we-can-take-road-trips-now-where-are-we-supposed-go-bathroom/.

U.S. Centers for Disease Control and Prevention. "Considerations for Public Beaches." Centers for Disease Control and Prevention - Coronavirus Disease 2019 (COVID-19). Last modified June 16, 2020. Accessed July 14, 2020. https://www.cdc.gov/coronavirus/2019-ncov/community/parks-rec/public-beaches.html.

———. "Considerations for Public Pools, Hot Tubs, and Water Playgrounds During COVID-19." Centers for Disease Control and Prevention - Coronavirus Disease 2019 (COVID-19). Last modified May 27, 2020. Accessed July 14, 2020. https://www.cdc.gov/coronavirus/2019-ncov/community/parks-rec/aquatic-venues.html.

———. "Personal and Social Activities." Centers for Disease Control and Prevention - Coronavirus Disease 2019 (COVID-19). Last modified June 15, 2020. Accessed July 14, 2020. https://www.cdc.gov/coronavirus/2019-ncov/daily-life-coping/personal-social-activities.html.

———. "Suggestions for Youth and Summer Camps." Centers for Disease Control and Prevention - Coronavirus Disease 2019 (COVID-19). Last modified June 25, 2020. Accessed July 14, 2020. https://www.cdc.gov/coronavirus/2019-ncov/community/schools-childcare/summer-camps.html.

———. "Visiting Parks and Recreational Facilities." Centers for Disease Control and Prevention - Coronavirus Disease 2019 (COVID-19). Last modified June 9, 2020. Accessed July 14, 2020. https://www.cdc.gov/coronavirus/2019-ncov/daily-life-coping/visitors.html.

Xiao, Fei, Jing Sun, Yonghao Xu, Fang Li, Xiaofang Huang, Heying Li, Jingxian Zhao, Jicheng Huang, and Jincun Zhao. "Infectious SARS-CoV-2 in Feces of Patient with Severe COVID-19." *Emerging Infectious Diseases* 26, no. 8 (August 2020). Accessed July 14, 2020. https://doi.org/10.3201/eid2608.200681.

Family Guide to Covid

Al Jazeera. "Coronavirus: Lessons From Asia." May 3, 2020. Accessed June 4, 2020. https://www.aljazeera.com/programmes/specialseries/2020/05/coronavirus-lessons-asia-200501110507558.html.

Altmann, Daniel M., Daniel C. Douek, and Rosemary J. Boyton. "What policy makers need to know about COVID-19 protective immunity." *The Lancet* 395, no. 10236 (May 16, 2020): 1527-29. Accessed June 4, 2020. https://doi.org/10.1016/S0140-6736(20)30985-5.

American College of Obstetricians and Gynecologists. "Novel Coronavirus 2019 (COVID-19): Practical Advisory." ACOG Clinical. Last modified May 19, 2020. Accessed June 4, 2020. https://www.acog.org/clinical/clinical-guidance/practice-advisory/articles/2020/03/novel-coronavirus-2019.

American Diabetes Association. "How COVID-19 Impacts People with Diabetes." American Diabetes Association - COVID-19. Last modified 2020. Accessed June 4, 2020. https://www.diabetes.org/coronavirus-covid-19/how-coronavirus-impacts-people-with-diabetes.

———. "Planning for Coronavirus." American Diabetes Association - COVID-19. Last modified 2020. Accessed June 4, 2020. https://www.diabetes.org/coronavirus-covid-19/planning-for-coronavirus.

American Lung Association. "How Fast Is a Sneeze Versus a Cough? Cover Your Mouth Either Way!" Each Breath: A Blog by the American Lung Association. Last modified May 12, 2016. Accessed June 4, 2020. https://www.lung.org/blog/sneeze-versus-cough.

Appleby, Julie. "What Takes So Long? A Behind-The-Scenes Look At The Steps Involved In COVID-19 Testing." *Kaiser Health News*, May 30, 2020. Accessed June 4, 2020. https://khn.org/news/what-takes-so-long-a-behind-the-scenes-look-at-the-steps-involved-in-covid-19-testing/.

Associated Press. "Study suggests fetal coronavirus infection is possible." *Modern Healthcare*, July 10, 2020. Accessed July 14, 2020. https://www.modernhealthcare.com/safety-quality/study-suggests-fetal-coronavirus-infection-possible.

Avert. "COVID-19 and HIV." Avert: Global information and education on HIV and AIDS. Last modified June 3, 2020. Accessed June 4, 2020. https://www.avert.org/coronavirus/covid19-HIV.

Begley, Sharon. "What explains Covid-19's lethality for the elderly? Scientists look to 'twilight' of the immune system." *STAT News*, March 30, 2020. Accessed June 4, 2020. https://www.statnews.com/2020/03/30/what-explains-coronavirus-lethality-for-elderly/.

"Blood thinners being used to mitigate risk of clots in COVID-19 patients." CBS News. Last modified May 26, 2020. Accessed June 4, 2020.

https://www.cbsnews.com/news/coronavirus-blood-clots-covid-19-symptom-strokes-young-people/.

Blue Cross Blue Shield of Massachusetts. "Blue Cross Blue Shield of Massachusetts Processes 1 Million Telehealth Claims in 9 Weeks." Blue Cross Blue Shield of Massachusetts. Last modified May 21, 2020. Accessed June 4, 2020. http://newsroom.bluecrossma.com/2020-05-21-Blue-Cross-Blue-Shield-of-Massachusetts-Processes-1-Million-Telehealth-Claims-in-9-Weeks?utm_source=STAT+Newsletters&utm_campaign=ff37996f74-MR_COPY_01&utm_medium=email&utm_term=0_8cab1d7961-ff37996f74-151227717.

Branswell, Helen. "New reports raise possibility pregnant women can pass coronavirus to fetus, but risk is unclear." *STAT News*, March 26, 2020. Accessed July 14, 2020. https://www.statnews.com/2020/03/26/new-reports-raise-possibility-pregnant-women-can-pass-coronavirus-to-fetus-but-risk-is-unclear/.

Breslin, Noelle et.al. "Coronavirus disease 2019 infection among asymptomatic and symptomatic pregnant women: two weeks of confirmed presentations to an affiliated pair of New York City hospitals." *American Journal of Obstetrics & Gynecology MFM* 2, no. 2 (April 9, 2020). https://doi.org/10.1016/j.ajogmf.2020.100118.

Cai, Xiaofang, Yaoling Ma, Songbo Li, Yan Chen, Zhihui Rong, and Wenbin Li. "Clinical Characteristics of 5 COVID-19 Cases With Non-respiratory

Symptoms as the First Manifestation in Children." *Frontiers in Pediatrics*, May 12, 2020. Accessed June 4, 2020. https://doi.org/10.3389/fped.2020.00258.

California State Government. "Stay home Q&A." Covid19.CA.gov. Last modified June 4, 2020. Accessed June 4, 2020. https://covid19.ca.gov/stay-home-except-for-essential-needs/?campaign_id=49&emc=edit_ca_20200501&instance_id=18134&nl=california-today&regi_id=78159988&segment_id=26374&te=1&user_id=930b2d6d81 5949d1bd3f3835944a4f18#outdoor.

Campbell, Denis. "Quarter of Covid-19 deaths in English hospitals were of diabetics." *The Guardian*, May 14, 2020. Accessed June 4, 2020. https://www.theguardian.com/world/2020/may/14/one-in-four-people-who-died-in-uk-hospitals-with-covid-19-had-diabetes.

Cariou, B., Hadjadj, S., Wargny, M. et.al. "Phenotypic characteristics and prognosis of inpatients with COVID-19 and diabetes: the CORONADO study." *Diabetologia*, May 29, 2020. https://doi.org/10.1007/s00125-020-05180-x.

Carroll, Aaron E. "When Can Grandparents Meet the Newborn?" *New York Times*, June 16, 2020. Accessed July 14, 2020. https://www.nytimes.com/2020/06/16/parenting/baby/grandparents-meet-newborn-coronavirus.html.

Centers for Disease Control and Prevention. "CDC Releases Interim Reopening Guidance for Dental Settings." Centers for Disease Control and Prevention - Oral Health. Last modified June 3, 2020. Accessed June 4, 2020. https://www.cdc.gov/oralhealth/infectioncontrol/statement-COVID.html.

———. "Community Transmission of SARS-CoV-2 at Two Family Gatherings — Chicago, Illinois, February–March 2020." Morbidity and Mortality Weekly Report (MMWR). Last modified April 17, 2020. Accessed June 4, 2020. https://www.cdc.gov/mmwr/volumes/69/wr/mm6915e1.htm?s_cid=mm6915e1_w.

———. "Effects of the COVID-19 Pandemic on Routine Pediatric Vaccine Ordering and Administration — United States, 2020." Morbidity and Mortality Weekly Report (MMWR). Last modified May 15, 2020. Accessed June 4, 2020. https://www.cdc.gov/mmwr/volumes/69/wr/mm6919e2.htm.

———. "Evaluation and Management Considerations for Neonates At Risk for COVID-19." Centers for Disease Control and Prevention - Coronavirus Disease 2019 (COVID-19). Last modified May 20, 2020. Accessed July 14, 2020. https://www.cdc.gov/coronavirus/2019-ncov/hcp/caring-for-newborns.html.

———. "For Parents: Multisystem Inflammatory Syndrome in Children (MIS-C) associated with COVID-19." Centers for Disease Control and Prevention

- Coronavirus Disease 2019 (COVID-19). https://www.cdc.gov/coronavirus/2019-ncov/daily-life-coping/children/misc.html.

———. "Frequently Asked Questions." Centers for Disease Control and Prevention - Coronavirus Disease 2019 (COVID-19). Last modified June 2, 2020. Accessed June 4, 2020. https://www.cdc.gov/coronavirus/2019-ncov/faq.html.

———. "Groups at Higher Risk for Severe Illness." Centers for Disease Control and Prevention - Coronavirus Disease 2019 (COVID-19). Last modified May 14, 2020. Accessed June 4, 2020. https://www.cdc.gov/coronavirus/2019-ncov/need-extra-precautions/groups-at-higher-risk.html.

———. "Guidance for Child Care Programs that Remain Open." Centers for Disease Control and Prevention - Coronavirus Disease 2019 (COVID-19). Last modified April 21, 2020. Accessed June 4, 2020. https://www.cdc.gov/coronavirus/2019-ncov/community/schools-childcare/guidance-for-childcare.html.

———. "Hospitalization Rates and Characteristics of Patients Hospitalized with Laboratory-Confirmed Coronavirus Disease 2019 — COVID-NET, 14 States, March 1–30, 2020." Morbidity and Mortality Weekly Report (MMWR). Last modified April 17, 2020. Accessed June 4, 2020.

https://www.cdc.gov/mmwr/volumes/69/wr/mm6915e3.htm?s_cid=mm6915e3_w.

———. "How COVID-19 Spreads." Centers for Disease Control and Prevention - Coronavirus Disease 2019 (COVID-19). Last modified June 1, 2020. Accessed June 4, 2020. https://www.cdc.gov/coronavirus/2019-ncov/prevent-getting-sick/how-covid-spreads.html.

———. "How to Protect Yourself & Others." Centers for Disease Control and Prevention - Coronavirus Disease 2019 (COVID-19). Last modified April 24, 2020. Accessed June 4, 2020. https://www.cdc.gov/coronavirus/2019-ncov/prevent-getting-sick/prevention.html.

———. "If You Are Immunocompromised, Protect Yourself From COVID-19." Centers for Disease Control and Prevention - Coronavirus Disease 2019 (COVID-19). Last modified May 14, 2020. Accessed June 4, 2020. https://www.cdc.gov/coronavirus/2019-ncov/need-extra-precautions/immunocompromised.html.

———. "People of Any Age with Underlying Medical Conditions." Centers for Disease Control and Prevention - Coronavirus Disease 2019 (COVID-19). Last modified June 25, 2020. Accessed July 14, 2020. https://www.cdc.gov/coronavirus/2019-ncov/need-extra-precautions/people-with-medical-conditions.html.

————. "People Who Are at Increased Risk for Severe Illness." Centers for Disease Control and Prevention - Coronavirus Disease 2019 (COVID-19). Last modified June 25, 2020. Accessed July 14, 2020. https://www.cdc.gov/coronavirus/2019-ncov/need-extra-precautions/people-at-increased-risk.html?CDC_AA_refVal=https%3A%2F%2Fwww.cdc.gov%2Fcoronavirus%2F2019-ncov%2Fneed-extra-precautions%2Fpeople-at-higher-risk.html.

————. "People with Disabilities." Centers for Disease Control and Prevention - Coronavirus Disease 2019 (COVID-19). Last modified April 7, 2020. Accessed June 4, 2020. https://www.cdc.gov/coronavirus/2019-ncov/need-extra-precautions/people-with-disabilities.html.

————. "Personal Protective Equipment: Questions and Answers." Centers for Disease Control and Prevention - Coronavirus Disease 2019 (COVID-19). Last modified March 14, 2020. Accessed June 4, 2020. https://www.cdc.gov/coronavirus/2019-ncov/hcp/respirator-use-faq.html.

————. "Quarantine and isolation." Centers for Disease Control and Prevention - Quarantine and Isolation. Last modified September 29, 2017. Accessed July 14, 2020. https://www.cdc.gov/quarantine/index.html.

————. "Running Essential Errands." Centers for Disease Control and Prevention - Coronavirus Disease 2019 (COVID-19). Last modified May 11, 2020. Accessed June 4, 2020. https://www.cdc.gov/coronavirus/2019-ncov/daily-life-coping/essential-goods-services.html.

————. "Strategies to Optimize the Supply of PPE and Equipment." Centers for Disease Control and Prevention - Coronavirus Disease 2019 (COVID-19). Last modified May 18, 2020. Accessed June 4, 2020. https://www.cdc.gov/coronavirus/2019-ncov/hcp/ppe-strategy/index.html.

————. "Vaccination of Tier 1 at All Pandemic Severities." Centers for Disease Control and Prevention - Influenza (Flu). Last modified October 24, 2018. Accessed May 29, 2020. https://www.cdc.gov/flu/pandemic-resources/national-strategy/planning-guidance/pandemic-severities-tier-1.html.

————. "Visiting Parks and Recreational Facilities." Centers for Disease Control and Prevention - Coronavirus Disease 2019 (COVID-19). Last modified May 19, 2020. Accessed June 4, 2020. https://www.cdc.gov/coronavirus/2019-ncov/daily-life-coping/visitors.html.

————. "What You Can Do." Centers for Disease Control and Prevention - Coronavirus Disease 2019 (COVID-19). Last modified May 8, 2020. Accessed June 4, 2020. https://www.cdc.gov/coronavirus/2019-ncov/need-extra-precautions/what-you-can-do.html.

————. "When You Can be Around Others After You Had or Likely Had COVID-19." Centers for Disease Control and Prevention - Coronavirus Disease 2019 (COVID-19). Last modified May 26, 2020. Accessed July 14, 2020. https://www.cdc.gov/coronavirus/2019-ncov/if-you-are-sick/end-home-isolation.html.

Cha, Ariana Eunjung. "Young and middle-aged people, barely sick with covid-19, are dying of strokes." *Washington Post*, April 25, 2020. Accessed June 4, 2020. https://www.washingtonpost.com/health/2020/04/24/strokes-coronavirus-young-patients/.

Cha, Ariana Eunjung, and Chelsea Janes. "Young adults are also affected by Kawasaki-like disease linked to coronavirus, doctors say." *Washington Post*, May 21, 2020. Accessed June 4, 2020. https://www.washingtonpost.com/health/2020/05/21/misc-c-kawasaki-coronavirus-young-adults/.

Chee, Ying Jie, Shereen Jia Huey, and Ester Yeoha. "Diabetic ketoacidosis precipitated by Covid-19 in a patient with newly diagnosed diabetes mellitus." *Diabetes Research and Clinical Practice*, April 24, 2020. Accessed July 14, 2020. https://doi.org/10.1016/j.diabres.2020.108166.

Cirillo, Francesco. "The Pomodoro Technique®." The Pomodoro Technique®. Last modified 2020. Accessed June 4, 2020. https://francescocirillo.com/pages/pomodoro-technique.

Cohen, Joshua. "The Complex Global Evolution Of Coronavirus Mask Rules." *Forbes*, July 12, 2020. Accessed July 14, 2020. https://www.forbes.com/sites/joshuacohen/2020/07/12/the-complex-global-evolution-of--coronavirus-mask-rules/#868b5ed428d2.

Coombs, Bertha. "Telehealth visits are booming as doctors and patients embrace distancing amid the coronavirus crisis." CNBC. Last modified April 4, 2020. Accessed June 4, 2020. https://www.cnbc.com/2020/04/03/telehealth-visits-could-top-1-billion-in-2020-amid-the-coronavirus-crisis.html.

Cullinane, Carl, and Rebecca Montacute. "COVID-19 and Social Mobility Impact Brief #1: School Shutdown." The Sutton Trust. Last modified April 2020. Accessed June 4, 2020. https://www.suttontrust.com/wp-content/uploads/2020/04/COVID-19-Impact-Brief-School-Shutdown.pdf.

David Ellinghaus et. al. "The ABO blood group locus and a chromosome 3 gene cluster associate with SARS-CoV-2 respiratory failure in an Italian-Spanish genome-wide association analysis." *medRxiv*, June 2, 2020. Accessed July 14, 2020. https://doi.org/10.1101/2020.05.31.20114991.

Dean, Natalie E. "COVID-19 Data Dives: Why Don't We Have a Vaccine for SARS or MERS?" *Medscape*, May 28, 2020. Accessed May 29, 2020. https://www.medscape.com/viewarticle/931226.

Dizik, Alina. "What We Know About Face Shields and Coronavirus." *Wall Street Journal*, June 16, 2020. Accessed July 14, 2020. https://www.wsj.com/articles/what-we-know-about-face-shields-and-coronavirus-11592321931?st=i4dcpazmkmnudz0&reflink=article_email_share.

"Does the flu vaccine work as well in elderly people?" *Harvard Health Publishing*, December 2019. Accessed May 29, 2020. https://www.health.harvard.edu/diseases-and-conditions/does-the-flu-vaccine-work-as-well-in-elderly-people.

Duan, Kai et.al. "The feasibility of convalescent plasma therapy in severe COVID-19 patients: a pilot study." *medRxiv*, March 23, 2020. Accessed May 29, 2020. https://doi.org/10.1101/2020.03.16.20036145.

Edmond J. Safra Center for Ethics at Harvard University. "Road to Pandemic Resilience." Edmond J. Safra Center for Ethics at Harvard University. Last modified April 20, 2020. Accessed June 4, 2020. https://ethics.harvard.edu/files/center-for-ethics/files/roadmaptopandemicresilience_updated_4.20.20_0.pdf.

Elizabeth J. Williamson et.al. "OpenSAFELY: factors associated with COVID-19 death in 17 million patients." *Nature*, July 8, 2020. Accessed July 14, 2020. https://doi.org/10.1038/s41586-020-2521-4.

European Lung Foundation. "Covid-19 and lung disease Q&A." European Lung Foundation - COVID-19. Last modified May 27, 2020. Accessed June 4, 2020. https://www.europeanlung.org/covid-19/covid-19-information-and-resources/covid-19-info.

Farge, Emma, and Michael Shields. "'This virus may never go away,' WHO says." *Reuters*, May 13, 2020. Accessed May 29, 2020.

https://www.reuters.com/article/us-health-coronavirus-who-briefing/this-virus-may-never-go-away-who-says-idUSKBN22P2IJ.

Forster, Victoria. "Wearing A Mask To Reduce The Spread Of Coronavirus Will Not Give You Carbon Dioxide Poisoning." *Forbes*, May 12, 2020. Accessed June 4, 2020. https://www.forbes.com/sites/victoriaforster/2020/05/12/wearing-a-mask-to-reduce-the-spread-of-coronavirus-will-not-give-you-carbon-dioxide-poisoning/#660a241017f5.

Fottrell, Quentin. "Black Americans are twice as likely to be hospitalized from COVID-19." MarketWatch. Last modified June 4, 2020. Accessed June 4, 2020. https://www.marketwatch.com/story/75-of-frontline-workers-in-new-york-the-epicenter-of-coronavirus-are-people-of-color-and-black-americans-are-twice-as-likely-to-die-from-covid-19-2020-06-01.

Franklin-Wallis, Oliver. "How School Shutdowns Have Long-Term Effects on Children." *WIRED UK*, May 18, 2020. Accessed June 4, 2020. https://www.wired.com/story/how-school-shutdowns-have-longterm-effects-on-children/?utm_source=onsite-share&utm_medium=email&utm_campaign=onsite-share&utm_brand=wired.

Gallagher, James. "Coronavirus cure: When will we have a drug to treat it?" *BBC News*, May 27, 2020. Accessed June 4, 2020. https://www.bbc.com/news/health-52354520.

Gostic, Katelyn, Ana CR Gomez, Riley O. Mummah, Adam J. Kucharski, and James O. Lloyd-Smith. "Estimated effectiveness of symptom and risk screening to prevent the spread of COVID-19." *eLife Sciences*, February 24, 2020. Accessed June 4, 2020. https://doi.org/10.7554/eLife.55570.

Hahn, Stephen M., and Jeffrey E. Shuren. "Coronavirus (COVID-19) Update: FDA Authorizes First Antigen Test to Help in the Rapid Detection of the Virus that Causes COVID-19 in Patients." U.S. Food & Drug Administration. Last modified May 9, 2020. Accessed June 4, 2020. https://www.fda.gov/news-events/press-announcements/coronavirus-covid-19-update-fda-authorizes-first-antigen-test-help-rapid-detection-virus-causes.

Harvard Health Publishing. "If you've been exposed to the coronavirus." Harvard Health Publishing. Last modified May 28, 2020. Accessed June 4, 2020. https://www.health.harvard.edu/diseases-and-conditions/if-youve-been-exposed-to-the-coronavirus.

Harwell, Drew. "Thermal scanners are the latest technology being deployed to detect the coronavirus. But they don't really work." *Washington Post*, May 11, 2020. Accessed June 4, 2020. https://www.washingtonpost.com/technology/2020/05/11/thermal-scanners-are-latest-technology-being-deployed-detect-coronavirus-they-dont-really-work/.

Haseltine, William A. "How Antibody Tests Can Be Used To Fight COVID-19." *Forbes*, April 6, 2020. Accessed June 4, 2020.

https://www.forbes.com/sites/williamhaseltine/2020/04/06/how-antibody-tests-can-be-used-to-fight-covid-19/#70c7b57a3904.

———. "Why America Is Losing to COVID-19." *Project Syndicate*, March 31, 2020. Accessed June 4, 2020. https://www.project-syndicate.org/commentary/united-states-covid-testing-contact-tracing-by-william-a-haseltine-2020-03.

He, X., Lau, E.H.Y., Wu, P. et.al. "Temporal dynamics in viral shedding and transmissibility of COVID-19." *Nature Medicine* 26 (April 15, 2020): 672-75. Accessed June 4, 2020. https://doi.org/10.1038/s41591-020-0869-5.

Hinde, Natasha. "Why Wearing Gloves To The Grocery Store Won't Protect You From COVID-19." HuffPost. Last modified June 2, 2020. Accessed June 4, 2020. https://www.huffpost.com/entry/wearing-gloves-to-grocery-store-coronavirus_l_5ed656abc5b63e9c88e4d4bc?utm_campaign=share_email&ncid=other_email_o63gt2jcad4.

Hogdson, Camilla. "Mystery of prolonged Covid-19 symptoms adds to unknowns." *Financial Times*, May 16, 2020. Accessed June 4, 2020. https://www.ft.com/content/91e4482e-d120-49ab-93e3-d314d99b5336.

Holdeman, Eric. "COVID-19: Transmission Scenarios Explained." *Government Technology*, May 11, 2020. Accessed June 4, 2020. https://www.govtech.com/em/emergency-blogs/disaster-zone/covid-19-transmission-scenarios-explained.html.

Hooper, Monica Webb, Anna María Nápoles, and Eliseo J. Pérez-Stable. "COVID-19 and Racial/Ethnic Disparities." *JAMA*, May 11, 2020. Accessed June 4, 2020. https://doi.org/10.1001/jama.2020.8598.

Huang, Yasheng, Meicen Sun, and Yuze Sui. "How Digital Contact Tracing Slowed Covid-19 in East Asia." *Harvard Business Review*, April 15, 2020. Accessed June 4, 2020. https://hbr.org/2020/04/how-digital-contact-tracing-slowed-covid-19-in-east-asia.

Huijun Chen et.al. "Clinical characteristics and intrauterine vertical transmission potential of COVID-19 infection in nine pregnant women: a retrospective review of medical records." *The Lancet* 395, no. 10226 (February 12, 2020): 809-15. Accessed July 14, 2020. https://doi.org/10.1016/S0140-6736(20)30360-3.

Hung, Ivan Fan-Ngai et.al. "Triple combination of interferon beta-1b, lopinavir–ritonavir, and ribavirin in the treatment of patients admitted to hospital with COVID-19: an open-label, randomised, phase 2 trial." *The Lancet* 395, no. 10238 (May 30, 2020): 1695-704. Accessed May 29, 2020. https://doi.org/10.1016/S0140-6736(20)31042-4.

International Chronic Myeloid Leukemia Foundation. "Advice for people with Chronic Myeloid Leukemia on COVID-19 (coronavirus)." International Chronic Myeloid Leukemia Foundation. Last modified March 2020. Accessed June 4, 2020. https://www.cml-foundation.org/news-icmlf-mobile/1437-

advice-for-people-with-chronic-myeloid-leukemia-on-covid-19-coronavirus.html.

International Society for Infectious Diseases. "An update letter from the Minister of Agriculture to the Dutch House of Representatives." Program for Monitoring Emerging Diseases. Last modified May 25, 2020. Accessed June 4, 2020. https://promedmail.org/promed-post/?id=20200525.7375359.

Janes, Chelsea. "In some nations, government isolation centers helped reduce coronavirus infections. The U.S. has resisted the strategy." *Washington Post*, May 20, 2020. Accessed June 4, 2020. https://www.washingtonpost.com/health/in-some-nations-government-isolation-centers-helped-reduce-covid-19-infections-the-us-has-resisted-the-strategy/2020/05/19/533850d6-9616-11ea-9f5e-56d8239bf9ad_story.html.

Jeffrey Seow et.al. "Longitudinal evaluation and decline of antibody responses in SARS-CoV-2 infection." *medRxiv*, July 11, 2020. Accessed July 14, 2020. https://doi.org/10.1101/2020.07.09.20148429.

Joseph, Andrew. "CDC: Some Americans are misusing cleaning products — including drinking them — in effort to kill coronavirus." STAT News. Last modified June 5, 2020. Accessed July 14, 2020. https://www.statnews.com/2020/06/05/cdc-misusing-bleach-try-kill-coronavirus/.

Khan, Amir. "Doctor's Note: What are serology tests and do they work?" *Al Jazeera*, May 9, 2020. Accessed June 4, 2020. https://www.aljazeera.com/indepth/features/doctor-note-serology-tests-work-200505151942226.html.

King, Anthony. "What four coronaviruses from history can tell us about covid-19." *New Scientist*, April 29, 2020. Accessed June 4, 2020. https://www.newscientist.com/article/mg24632800-700-what-four-coronaviruses-from-history-can-tell-us-about-covid-19/.

Kirkcaldy, Robert D., Brian A. King, and John T. Brooks. "COVID-19 and Postinfection Immunity: Limited Evidence, Many Remaining Questions." *JAMA*, May 11, 2020. Accessed June 4, 2020. https://doi.org/10.1001/jama.2020.7869.

Koran, Mario. "'It's irresponsible': Washington state warns against 'coronavirus parties.'" *The Guardian*, May 6, 2020. Accessed June 4, 2020. https://www.theguardian.com/world/2020/may/06/its-irresponsible-washington-state-sees-sudden-rise-in-covid-parties.

Landi, Heather. "Half of physicians now using telehealth as COVID-19 changes practice operations." *Fierce Healthcare*, April 23, 2020. Accessed June 4, 2020. https://www.fiercehealthcare.com/practices/half-physicians-now-using-telehealth-as-covid-changes-practice-operations.

Lanese, Nicoletta. "First at-home saliva test for COVID-19 earns FDA approval." Live Science. Last modified May 2020. Accessed June 4, 2020. https://www.livescience.com/at-home-saliva-test-for-covid19.html.

Lazar, Kay, and Andrew Ryan. "No, warm weather will not kill the coronavirus." *Boston Globe*, April 24, 2020. Accessed June 4, 2020. https://www.bostonglobe.com/2020/04/24/nation/no-warm-weather-will-not-kill-coronavirus/.

Lee, Bruce Y. "Where Coronavirus Is More Likely To Be Airborne, 5 Places To Avoid." *Forbes*, May 30, 2020. Accessed June 4, 2020. https://www.forbes.com/sites/brucelee/2020/05/30/where-coronavirus-is-more-likely-to-be-airborne-5-places-to-avoid/#44f194bb39ab.

Leffler, David. "Coronavirus placing high stress on new, expecting moms and raising risks for mental health issues." *Washington Post*, June 21, 2020. Accessed July 14, 2020. https://www.washingtonpost.com/health/coronavirus-placing-high-stress-on-new-expecting-moms-and-raising-risks-for-mental-health-issues/2020/06/18/1f5649c6-aa66-11ea-a9d9-a81c1a491c52_story.html.

Li, Diangeng, Meiling Jin, and Pengtao Bao. "Clinical Characteristics and Results of Semen Tests Among Men With Coronavirus Disease 2019." *JAMA Network Open* 3, no. 5 (May 7, 2020). Accessed June 4, 2020. https://doi.org/10.1001/jamanetworkopen.2020.8292.

Li, Yun-yun, Ji-Xiang Wang, and Xi Chen. "Can a toilet promote virus transmission? From a fluid dynamics perspective." *Physics of Fluids*, June 16, 2020. Accessed July 14, 2020. https://doi.org/10.1063/5.0013318.

Lippi, Giuseppe. "Chronic obstructive pulmonary disease is associated with severe coronavirus disease 2019 (COVID-19)." *Respiratory Medicine*, June 2020. https://doi.org/10.1016/j.rmed.2020.105941.

Li, W., Wang, D., Guo, J. et.al. "COVID-19 in persons with chronic myeloid leukaemia." *Leukemia*, May 18, 2020. Accessed June 4, 2020. https://doi.org/10.1038/s41375-020-0853-6.

Mallapaty, Smriti. "Mounting clues suggest the coronavirus might trigger diabetes." *Nature*, June 24, 2020. Accessed July 14, 2020. https://www.nature.com/articles/d41586-020-01891-8.

———. "What's the risk that animals will spread the coronavirus?" *Nature*, June 1, 2020. Accessed June 4, 2020. https://www.nature.com/articles/d41586-020-01574-4?utm_source=Nature+Briefing&utm_campaign=32981e1f33-briefing-dy-20200601&utm_medium=email&utm_term=0_c9dfd39373-32981e1f33-45423538.

Mandavilli, Apoorva. "Airborne Coronavirus: What You Should Do Now." *New York Times*, July 6, 2020. Accessed July 14, 2020.

https://www.nytimes.com/2020/07/06/health/coronavirus-airborne-aerosols.html?smid=em-share.

———. "New Studies Add to Evidence that Children May Transmit the Coronavirus." *New York Times*, May 8, 2020. Accessed June 4, 2020. https://www.nytimes.com/2020/05/05/health/coronavirus-children-transmission-school.html?smid=em-share.

———. "239 Experts With One Big Claim: The Coronavirus Is Airborne." *New York Times*, July 4, 2020. Accessed July 14, 2020. https://www.nytimes.com/2020/07/04/health/239-experts-with-one-big-claim-the-coronavirus-is-airborne.html.

March of Dimes. "Coronavirus Disease (COVID-19): What You Need to Know About Its Impact on Moms and Babies." March of Dimes. Last modified May 29, 2020. Accessed June 4, 2020. https://www.marchofdimes.org/complications/coronavirus-disease-covid-19-what-you-need-to-know.aspx.

McCray, Eugene, and Jonathan H. Mermin. "PrEP During COVID-19." Centers for Disease Control and Prevention - National Center for HIV/AIDS, Viral Hepatitis, STD, and TB Prevention. Last modified May 15, 2020. Accessed June 4, 2020. https://www.cdc.gov/nchhstp/dear_colleague/2020/dcl-051520-PrEP-during-COVID-19.html.

Mehrotra, Ateev, Michael Chernew, David Linetsky, David Cutler, and Hilary Hatch. "The Impact of the COVID-19 Pandemic on Outpatient Visits: A Rebound Emerges." The Commonwealth Fund. Last modified May 19, 2020. Accessed June 4, 2020. https://www.commonwealthfund.org/publications/2020/apr/impact-covid-19-outpatient-visits.

Metzger, Kylene. "Slow the Spread with Cloth Masks." University of Utah Health Feed Blog. Last modified May 6, 2020. Accessed June 4, 2020. https://healthcare.utah.edu/healthfeed/postings/2020/03/coronavirus-face-masks.php.

Muenter, Olivia. "How Often You Should Wash Your Sheets During The Coronavirus Pandemic." HuffPost. Last modified May 5, 2020. https://www.huffpost.com/entry/how-often-wash-sheets-coronavirus-pandemic_l_5eac4f6bc5b624b396929d10?utm_campaign=share_email&ncid=other_email_o63gt2jcad4.

Nadia Oreshkova et.al. "SARS-CoV2 infection in farmed mink, Netherlands, April 2020." *bioRxiv*, May 18, 2020. Accessed June 4, 2020. https://doi.org/10.1101/2020.05.18.101493.

National Cancer Research Institute. "COVID-19 (coronavirus) advice for patients with Chronic Myeloid Leukaemia receiving TKI therapy." British Society for Haematology. Last modified March 21, 2020. Accessed June 4,

2020.   https://b-s-h.org.uk/media/18154/covid-19-and-cml-recommendations-ncri-sub-group-21_3_20.pdf.

National Institutes of Health. "COVID-19, MERS & SARS." National Institute of Allergy and Infectious Diseases - Coronavirus. Last modified April 6, 2020. Accessed   July   14,   2020.   https://www.niaid.nih.gov/diseases-conditions/covid-19.

————. "NIAID Emerging Infectious Diseases/ Pathogens." National Institute of Allergy and Infectious Disease - Biodefense. Last modified July 26, 2018. Accessed   June   4,   2020.   https://www.niaid.nih.gov/research/emerging-infectious-diseases-pathogens.

Neeltje van Doremalen et.al. "Aerosol and Surface Stability of SARS-CoV-2 as Compared With SARS-CoV-1." *New England Journal of Medicine* 382, no. 16 (April 16, 2020). https://doi.org/10.1056/NEJMc2004973.

NYU Shanghai. "NYU Shanghai to Begin Reopening to Students April 27." NYU Shanghai. Last modified April 24, 2020. Accessed June 4, 2020. https://shanghai.nyu.edu/news/nyu-shanghai-begin-reopening-students-april-27.

Omar Abdel-Mannan et.al. "Neurologic and Radiographic Findings Associated With COVID-19 Infection in Children." *JAMA Neurology*, July 1, 2020.   Accessed   July   14,   2020. https://doi.org/10.1001/jamaneurol.2020.2687.

Paranjpe, Ishan et.al. "Association of Treatment Dose Anticoagulation with In-Hospital Survival Among Hospitalized Patients with COVID-19." *Journal of the American College of Cardiology*, May 6, 2020. Accessed May 29, 2020. https://doi.org/10.1016/j.jacc.2020.05.001.

Parker-Pope, Tara. "Have I Been Cleaning All Wrong?" *New York Times*, May 13, 2020. Accessed June 4, 2020. https://www.nytimes.com/2020/05/06/well/live/coronavirus-cleaning-cleaners-disinfectants-home.html?smid=em-share.

Patel, Ami, Mamadou A. Bah, and David B. Weiner. "In Vivo Delivery of Nucleic Acid-Encoded Monoclonal Antibodies." *BioDrugs* 34 (March 10, 2020): 273-93. https://doi.org/10.1007/s40259-020-00412-3.

Patel, Neel V. "Antigen testing could be a faster, cheaper way to diagnose covid-19." *MIT Technology Review*, April 24, 2020. Accessed June 4, 2020. https://www.technologyreview.com/2020/04/24/1000486/antigen-testing-could-faster-cheaper-diagnose-covid-19-coronavirus/.

Paton, James, Jason Gale, and John Lauerman. "The Race to Develop a Coronavirus Vaccine: What you need to know." *Bloomberg*, May 8, 2020. Accessed May 29, 2020. https://www.bloomberg.com/news/storythreads/2020-05-08/the-race-to-develop-a-coronavirus-vaccine.

Pesheva, Ekaterina. "Outpatient COVID-19 Clues." Harvard Medical School - News & Research. Last modified May 6, 2020. Accessed June 4, 2020. https://hms.harvard.edu/news/outpatient-covid-19-clues#.Xrp8gJ_9h4c.mailto.

Pizzorno, Andrés, Blandine Padey, Olivier Terrier, and Manuel Rosa-Calatrava. "Drug Repurposing Approaches for the Treatment of Influenza Viral Infection: Reviving Old Drugs to Fight Against a Long-Lived Enemy." *Frontiers in Immunology* 10, no. 531 (March 19, 2020). Accessed May 29, 2020. https://doi.org/10.3389/fimmu.2019.00531.

Quan-Xin Long et.al. "Clinical and immunological assessment of asymptomatic SARS-CoV-2 infections." *Nature Medicine*, June 18, 2020. Accessed July 14, 2020. https://doi.org/10.1038/s41591-020-0965-6.

Rabin, Roni Caryn. "What Is 'Covid Toe'? Maybe a Strange Sign of Coronavirus Infection." *New York Times*, May 5, 2020. Accessed June 4, 2020. https://www.nytimes.com/2020/05/01/health/coronavirus-covid-toe.html?smid=em-share.

Reynolds, Harmony et.al. "Renin–Angiotensin–Aldosterone System Inhibitors and Risk of Covid-19." *New England Journal of Medicine*, May 1, 2020. Accessed June 4, 2020. https://doi.org/10.1056/NEJMoa2008975.

Rogers, Adam. "How Does a Virus Spread in Cities? It's a Problem of Scale." *WIRED*, May 20, 2020. Accessed June 4, 2020.

https://www.wired.com/story/how-does-a-virus-spread-in-cities-its-a-problem-of-scale/.

Ross W Paterson et.al. "The emerging spectrum of COVID-19 neurology: clinical, radiological and laboratory findings." *Brain*, July 8, 2020. Accessed July 14, 2020. https://doi.org/10.1093/brain/awaa240.

Sascha Ellington et.al. "Characteristics of Women of Reproductive Age with Laboratory-Confirmed SARS-CoV-2 Infection by Pregnancy Status — United States, January 22–June 7, 2020." Morbidity and Mortality Weekly Report (MMWR). Last modified June 26, 2020. Accessed July 14, 2020. https://www.cdc.gov/mmwr/volumes/69/wr/mm6925a1.htm.

Schoch, Deborah. "amilies Anxious Over Loved Ones in Nursing Homes, Assisted Living." AARP Resources for Caregivers. Last modified April 2, 2020. Accessed June 4, 2020. https://www.aarp.org/caregiving/health/info-2020/preventing-coronavirus-in-nursing-homes.html.

The Scripps Research Institute. "Mutated coronavirus shows significant boost in infectivity." Scripps Research. Last modified June 12, 2020. Accessed July 14, 2020. https://www.scripps.edu/news-and-events/press-room/2020/20200612-choe-farzan-coronavirus-spike-mutation.html.

Sia, S.F., Yan, L., Chin, A.W.H. et.al. "Pathogenesis and transmission of SARS-CoV-2 in golden hamsters." *Nature*, May 14, 2020. Accessed June 4, 2020. https://doi.org/10.1038/s41586-020-2342-5.

Spinelli, Alexander. "Recovery from Covid-19 is filled with uncertainty. An antibody test offered me a little comfort." *STAT News*, May 21, 2020. Accessed June 4, 2020. https://www.statnews.com/2020/05/21/recovery-from-covid-19-antibodies-uncertainty/.

Stadnytskyi, Valentyn, Christina E. Bax, Adriaan Bax, and Philip Anfinrud. "The airborne lifetime of small speech droplets and their potential importance in SARS-CoV-2 transmission." *Proceedings of the National Academy of Sciences of the United States of America* 117, no. 22 (May 13, 2020): 11875-77. Accessed June 4, 2020. https://doi.org/10.1073/pnas.2006874117.

Teitell, Beth. "We can take road trips now. But where are we supposed to go to the bathroom?" *Boston Globe*, June 8, 2020. Accessed July 14, 2020. https://www.bostonglobe.com/2020/06/08/nation/we-can-take-road-trips-now-where-are-we-supposed-go-bathroom/.

University of Oxford. "Co-SPACE study - COVID-19: Supporting Parents, Adolescents, and Children during Epidemics." Department of Experimental Psychology at University of Oxford. Accessed June 4, 2020. https://oxfordxpsy.az1.qualtrics.com/jfe/form/SV_3VO130LTKOcloMd.

U.S. Food & Drug Administration. "Coronavirus (COVID-19) Update: FDA Issues Warning Letters to Companies Inappropriately Marketing Antibody Tests, Potentially Placing Public Health at Risk." FDA Newsroom. Last modified June 17, 2020. Accessed July 14, 2020. https://www.fda.gov/news-events/press-announcements/coronavirus-covid-19-update-fda-issues-warning-letters-companies-inappropriately-marketing-antibody.

———. "FDA COMBATING COVID-19 WITH THERAPEUTICS." U.S. Food & Drug Administration. Last modified May 11, 2020. Accessed June 4, 2020. https://www.fda.gov/media/136832/download.

———. "Recommendations for Investigational COVID-19 Convalescent Plasma." U.S. Food & Drug Administration. Last modified May 1, 2020. Accessed May 29, 2020. https://www.fda.gov/vaccines-blood-biologics/investigational-new-drug-ind-or-device-exemption-ide-process-cber/recommendations-investigational-covid-19-convalescent-plasma.

Vastag, Brian, and Beth Mazur. "Researchers warn covid-19 could cause debilitating long-term illness in some patients." *Washington Post*, May 30, 2020. Accessed June 4, 2020. https://www.washingtonpost.com/health/could-covid-19-cause-long-term-chronic-fatigue-and-illness-in-some-patients/2020/05/29/bcd5edb2-a02c-11ea-b5c9-570a91917d8d_story.html.

Walker, Kate F., Keelin O'Donoghue, Nicky Grace, Jon Dorling, Jeannette L. Comeau, Wentao Li, and Jim G. Thornton. "Maternal transmission of SARS-COV-2 to the neonate, and possible routes for such transmission: A systematic review and critical analysis." *Search Results Web Result with Site Links BJOG: An International Journal of Obstetrics & Gynaecology*, June 12, 2020. Accessed July 14, 2020. https://doi.org/10.1111/1471-0528.16362.

Watson, Clare. "How countries are using genomics to help avoid a second coronavirus wave." *Nature*, May 27, 2020. Accessed June 4, 2020. https://www.nature.com/articles/d41586-020-01573-5.

Watterberg, Kristi, and COMMITTEE ON FETUS AND NEWBORN. "Providing Care for Infants Born at Home." *Pediatrics* 145, no. 5 (May 2020). Accessed June 4, 2020. https://doi.org/10.1542/peds.2020-0626.

Weigel, Gabriela, Amrutha Ramaswarmy, Laurie Sobel, Alina Salganicoff, Juliette Cubanski, and Meredith Freed. "Opportunities and Barriers for Telemedicine in the U.S. During the COVID-19 Emergency and Beyond." Kaiser Family Foundation - Women's Health Policy. Last modified May 11, 2020. Accessed June 4, 2020. https://www.kff.org/womens-health-policy/issue-brief/opportunities-and-barriers-for-telemedicine-in-the-u-s-during-the-covid-19-emergency-and-beyond/.

Willyard, Cassandra. "Coronavirus blood-clot mystery intensifies." *Nature*, May 8, 2020. Accessed June 4, 2020. https://www.nature.com/articles/d41586-020-01403-8.

Wilson, Jillian. "How To Sleep Better If Coronavirus Anxiety Is Keeping You Awake." HuffPost. Last modified April 9, 2020. Accessed June 4, 2020. https://www.huffpost.com/entry/sleep-better-coronavirus-anxiety_l_5e8b5b2cc5b6cc1e47799a4d.

World Health Organization. "Advice on the use of point-of-care immunodiagnostic tests for COVID-19." World Health Organization. Last modified April 8, 2020. Accessed June 4, 2020. https://www.who.int/news-room/commentaries/detail/advice-on-the-use-of-point-of-care-immunodiagnostic-tests-for-covid-19.

———. "Coronavirus disease 2019 (COVID-19) Situation Report – 73." World Health Organization. Last modified April 2, 2020. Accessed June 4, 2020. https://www.who.int/docs/default-source/coronaviruse/situation-reports/20200402-sitrep-73-covid-19.pdf.

———. "Report of the WHO-China Joint Mission on Coronavirus Disease 2019 (COVID-19)." World Health Organization. Last modified February 24, 2020. Accessed June 4, 2020. https://www.who.int/docs/default-source/coronaviruse/who-china-joint-mission-on-covid-19-final-report.pdf.

———. "WHO statement: Tobacco use and COVID-19." World Health Organization. Last modified May 11, 2020. Accessed June 4, 2020. https://www.who.int/news-room/detail/11-05-2020-who-statement-tobacco-use-and-covid-19.

World Organisation for Animal Health. "Questions and Answers on the COVID-19." OIE - World Organisation for Animal Health. Last modified May 26, 2020. Accessed June 4, 2020. https://www.oie.int/en/scientific-expertise/specific-information-and-recommendations/questions-and-answers-on-2019novel-coronavirus/.

Xiao, Fei, Jing Sun, Yonghao Xu, Fang Li, Xiaofang Huang, Heying Li, Jingxian Zhao, Jicheng Huang, and Jincun Zhao. "Infectious SARS-CoV-2 in Feces of Patient with Severe COVID-19." *Emerging Infectious Diseases* 26, no. 8 (August 2020). Accessed July 14, 2020. https://doi.org/10.3201/eid2608.200681.

Yong, Ed. "COVID-19 Can Last for Several Months." *The Atlantic*, June 4, 2020. Accessed July 14, 2020. https://www.theatlantic.com/health/archive/2020/06/covid-19-coronavirus-longterm-symptoms-months/612679/?utm_source=atl&utm_medium=email&utm_campaign=share.

Yuanyuan Dong et.al. "Epidemiology of COVID-19 Among Children in China." *Pediatrics* 145, no. 6 (June 2020). Accessed July 14, 2020. https://doi.org/10.1542/peds.2020-0702.

Zeng, Hui et.al. "Antibodies in Infants Born to Mothers With COVID-19 Pneumonia." *JAMA* 323, no. 18 (March 26, 2020): 1848-49. Accessed June 4, 2020. https://doi.org/10.1001/jama.2020.4861.

Zhou, Hong et.al. "A Novel Bat Coronavirus Closely Related to SARS-CoV-2 Contains Natural Insertions at the S1/S2 Cleavage Site of the Spike Protein." *Current Biology*, May 10, 2020. Accessed June 4, 2020. https://doi.org/10.1016/j.cub.2020.05.023.

ACKNOWLEDGEMENTS

Thank you to all of the colleagues and mentors I have worked with over the years in classrooms, laboratories and offices around the world.

I would especially like to thank my former Harvard colleagues in the department of HIV/AIDS research and the department of human retrovirology research, many of whom continue to find solutions for some of the most important infectious disease and public health challenges facing the world today. I thank them not only for the work they have done and continue to do, but also for their efforts to preserve and expand upon the knowledge they have gained by cultivating and training new generations of young scientists.

Finally, I would like to express my sincere appreciation to my colleagues at ACCESS Health International, including Anna Dirksen. I would especially like to thank Josephine Gurch, whose editorial support ensures that this living book keeps pace with our ever-changing reality.

[i] Centers for Disease Control and Prevention, "How to Protect Yourself & Others," Centers for Disease Control and Prevention - Coronavirus Disease 2019 (COVID-19), last modified April 24, 2020, accessed June 4, 2020, https://www.cdc.gov/coronavirus/2019-ncov/prevent-getting-sick/prevention.html.

[ii] Joshua Cohen, "The Complex Global Evolution Of Coronavirus Mask Rules," *Forbes*, July 12, 2020, accessed July 14, 2020, https://www.forbes.com/sites/joshuacohen/2020/07/12/the-complex-global-evolution-of--coronavirus-mask-rules/#868b5ed428d2.

[iii] Kylene Metzger, "Slow the Spread with Cloth Masks," University of Utah Health Feed Blog, last modified May 6, 2020, accessed June 4, 2020, https://healthcare.utah.edu/healthfeed/postings/2020/03/coronavirus-face-masks.php.

[iv] Alina Dizik, "What We Know About Face Shields and Coronavirus," *Wall Street Journal*, June 16, 2020, accessed July 14, 2020, https://www.wsj.com/articles/what-we-know-about-face-shields-and-coronavirus-11592321931?st=i4dcpazmkmnudz0&reflink=article_email_share.

[v] Victoria Forster, "Wearing A Mask To Reduce The Spread Of Coronavirus Will Not Give You Carbon Dioxide Poisoning," *Forbes*, May 12, 2020, accessed June 4, 2020, https://www.forbes.com/sites/victoriaforster/2020/05/12/wearing-a-mask-to-reduce-the-spread-of-coronavirus-will-not-give-you-carbon-dioxide-poisoning/#660a241017f5.

[vi] Natasha Hinde, "Why Wearing Gloves To The Grocery Store Won't Protect You From COVID-19," HuffPost, last modified June 2, 2020, accessed June 4, 2020, https://www.huffpost.com/entry/wearing-gloves-to-

grocery-store-coronavirus_l_5ed656abc5b63e9c88e4d4bc?utm_campaign=share_email&ncid=other_email_o63gt2jcad4.

vii Centers for Disease Control and Prevention, "Effects of the COVID-19 Pandemic on Routine Pediatric Vaccine Ordering and Administration — United States, 2020," Morbidity and Mortality Weekly Report (MMWR), last modified May 15, 2020, accessed June 4, 2020, https://www.cdc.gov/mmwr/volumes/69/wr/mm6919e2.htm.

viii Centers for Disease Control and Prevention, "Guidance for Child Care Programs that Remain Open," Centers for Disease Control and Prevention - Coronavirus Disease 2019 (COVID-19), last modified April 21, 2020, accessed June 4, 2020, https://www.cdc.gov/coronavirus/2019-ncov/community/schools-childcare/guidance-for-childcare.html.

ix Child Care Aware, "Information for Families on Health and Safety Measures," last modified May 13, 2020, accessed June 5, 2020, https://info.childcareaware.org/hubfs/Health And Safety Measures For Families.pdf

x Centers for Disease Control and Prevention, "CDC Releases Interim Reopening Guidance for Dental Settings," Centers for Disease Control and Prevention - Oral Health, last modified June 3, 2020, accessed June 4, 2020, https://www.cdc.gov/oralhealth/infectioncontrol/statement-COVID.html.

xi Tara Parker-Pope, "Have I Been Cleaning All Wrong?," *New York Times*, May 13, 2020, accessed June 4, 2020, https://www.nytimes.com/2020/05/06/well/live/coronavirus-cleaning-cleaners-disinfectants-home.html?smid=em-share.

xii Andrew Joseph, "CDC: Some Americans are misusing cleaning products — including drinking them — in effort to kill coronavirus," STAT News, last

modified June 5, 2020, accessed July 14, 2020,
https://www.statnews.com/2020/06/05/cdc-misusing-bleach-try-kill-coronavirus/.

[xiii] Olivia Muenter, "How Often You Should Wash Your Sheets During The Coronavirus Pandemic," HuffPost, last modified May 5, 2020,
https://www.huffpost.com/entry/how-often-wash-sheets-coronavirus-pandemic_l_5eac4f6bc5b624b396929d10?utm_campaign=share_email&ncid=other_email_o63gt2jcad4.

[xiv] World Health Organization, "Coronavirus disease," World Health Organization.

[xv] Deborah Schoch, "amilies Anxious Over Loved Ones in Nursing Homes, Assisted Living," AARP Resources for Caregivers, last modified April 2, 2020, accessed June 4, 2020, https://www.aarp.org/caregiving/health/info-2020/preventing-coronavirus-in-nursing-homes.html.

[xvi] Centers for Disease Control and Prevention, "People with Disabilities," Centers for Disease Control and Prevention - Coronavirus Disease 2019 (COVID-19), last modified April 7, 2020, accessed June 4, 2020, https://www.cdc.gov/coronavirus/2019-ncov/need-extra-precautions/people-with-disabilities.html.

[xvii] Centers for Disease Control and Prevention, "People Who Are at Increased Risk for Severe Illness," Centers for Disease Control and Prevention - Coronavirus Disease 2019 (COVID-19), last modified June 25, 2020, accessed July 14, 2020, https://www.cdc.gov/coronavirus/2019-ncov/need-extra-precautions/people-at-increased-risk.html?CDC_AA_refVal=https%3A%2F%2Fwww.cdc.gov%2Fcoronavirus%2F2019-ncov%2Fneed-extra-precautions%2Fpeople-at-higher-risk.html.

[xviii] David Ellinghaus et. al, "The ABO blood group locus and a chromosome 3 gene cluster associate with SARS-CoV-2 respiratory failure in an Italian-

Spanish genome-wide association analysis," *medRxiv*, June 2, 2020, accessed July 14, 2020, https://doi.org/10.1101/2020.05.31.20114991.

[xix] Monica Webb Hooper, Anna María Nápoles, and Eliseo J. Pérez-Stable, "COVID-19 and Racial/Ethnic Disparities," *JAMA*, May 11, 2020, accessed June 4, 2020, https://doi.org/10.1001/jama.2020.8598.

[xx] Centers for Disease Control and Prevention, "Hospitalization Rates and Characteristics of Patients Hospitalized with Laboratory-Confirmed Coronavirus Disease 2019 — COVID-NET, 14 States, March 1–30, 2020," Morbidity and Mortality Weekly Report (MMWR), last modified April 17, 2020, accessed June 4, 2020, https://www.cdc.gov/mmwr/volumes/69/wr/mm6915e3.htm?s_cid=mm6915e3_w.

[xxi] Quentin Fottrell, "Black Americans are twice as likely to be hospitalized from COVID-19," MarketWatch, last modified June 4, 2020, accessed June 4, 2020, https://www.marketwatch.com/story/75-of-frontline-workers-in-new-york-the-epicenter-of-coronavirus-are-people-of-color-and-black-americans-are-twice-as-likely-to-die-from-covid-19-2020-06-01.

[xxii] Elizabeth J. Williamson et.al, "OpenSAFELY: factors associated with COVID-19 death in 17 million patients," *Nature*, July 8, 2020, accessed July 14, 2020, https://doi.org/10.1038/s41586-020-2521-4.

[xxiii] World Health Organization, "Coronavirus disease 2019 (COVID-19) Situation Report – 73," World Health Organization, last modified April 2, 2020, accessed June 4, 2020, https://www.who.int/docs/default-source/coronaviruse/situation-reports/20200402-sitrep-73-covid-19.pdf.

[xxiv] He, X., Lau, E.H.Y., Wu, P. et.al, "Temporal dynamics in viral shedding and transmissibility of COVID-19," *Nature Medicine* 26 (April 15, 2020, accessed June 4, 2020, https://doi.org/10.1038/s41591-020-0869-5.

[xxv] Centers for Disease Control and Prevention, "How COVID-19 Spreads," Centers for Disease Control and Prevention - Coronavirus Disease 2019 (COVID-19), last modified June 1, 2020, accessed June 4, 2020, https://www.cdc.gov/coronavirus/2019-ncov/prevent-getting-sick/how-covid-spreads.html.

[xxvi] Neeltje van Doremalen et.al, "Aerosol and Surface Stability of SARS-CoV-2 as Compared With SARS-CoV-1," *New England Journal of Medicine* 382, no. 16 (April 16, 2020), https://doi.org/10.1056/NEJMc2004973.

[xxvii] Centers for Disease Control and Prevention, "Frequently Asked Questions," Centers for Disease Control and Prevention - Coronavirus Disease 2019 (COVID-19), last modified June 2, 2020, accessed June 4, 2020, https://www.cdc.gov/coronavirus/2019-ncov/faq.html.

[xxviii] World Health Organization, "Report of the WHO-China Joint Mission on Coronavirus Disease 2019 (COVID-19)," World Health Organization, last modified February 24, 2020, accessed June 4, 2020, https://www.who.int/docs/default-source/coronaviruse/who-china-joint-mission-on-covid-19-final-report.pdf.

[xxix] Apoorva Mandavilli, "239 Experts With One Big Claim: The Coronavirus Is Airborne," *New York Times*, July 4, 2020, accessed July 14, 2020, https://www.nytimes.com/2020/07/04/health/239-experts-with-one-big-claim-the-coronavirus-is-airborne.html.

[xxx] American Lung Association, "How Fast Is a Sneeze Versus a Cough? Cover Your Mouth Either Way!," Each Breath: A Blog by the American Lung Association, last modified May 12, 2016, accessed June 4, 2020, https://www.lung.org/blog/sneeze-versus-cough.

[xxxi] Valentyn Stadnytskyi et al., "The airborne lifetime of small speech droplets and their potential importance in SARS-CoV-2

transmission," *Proceedings of the National Academy of Sciences of the United States of America* 117, no. 22 (May 13, 2020): [Page #], accessed June 4, 2020, https://doi.org/10.1073/pnas.2006874117.

xxxii Apoorva Mandavilli, "Airborne Coronavirus: What You Should Do Now," *New York Times*, July 6, 2020, accessed July 14, 2020, https://www.nytimes.com/2020/07/06/health/coronavirus-airborne-aerosols.html?smid=em-share.

xxxiii Stadnytskyi et al., "The airborne".

xxxiv Fei Xiao et al., "Infectious SARS-CoV-2 in Feces of Patient with Severe COVID-19," *Emerging Infectious Diseases* 26, no. 8 (August 2020), accessed July 14, 2020, https://doi.org/10.3201/eid2608.200681.

xxxv Yun-yun Li, Ji-Xiang Wang, and Xi Chen, "Can a toilet promote virus transmission? From a fluid dynamics perspective," *Physics of Fluids*, June 16, 2020, accessed July 14, 2020, https://doi.org/10.1063/5.0013318.

xxxvi Adam Rogers, "How Does a Virus Spread in Cities? It's a Problem of Scale," *WIRED*, May 20, 2020, accessed June 4, 2020, https://www.wired.com/story/how-does-a-virus-spread-in-cities-its-a-problem-of-scale/.

xxxvii Anthony King, "What four coronaviruses from history can tell us about covid-19," *New Scientist*, April 29, 2020, accessed June 4, 2020, https://www.newscientist.com/article/mg24632800-700-what-four-coronaviruses-from-history-can-tell-us-about-covid-19/.

xxxviii Apoorva Mandavilli, "New Studies Add to Evidence that Children May Transmit the Coronavirus," *New York Times*, May 8, 2020, accessed June 4, 2020, https://www.nytimes.com/2020/05/05/health/coronavirus-children-transmission-school.html?smid=em-share.

xxxix Smriti Mallapaty, "What's the risk that animals will spread the coronavirus?," *Nature*, June 1, 2020, accessed June 4, 2020, https://www.nature.com/articles/d41586-020-01574-4?utm_source=Nature+Briefing&utm_campaign=32981e1f33-briefing-dy-20200601&utm_medium=email&utm_term=0_c9dfd39373-32981e1f33-45423538.

xl World Organisation for Animal Health, "Questions and Answers on the COVID-19," OIE - World Organisation for Animal Health, last modified May 26, 2020, accessed June 4, 2020, https://www.oie.int/en/scientific-expertise/specific-information-and-recommendations/questions-and-answers-on-2019novel-coronavirus/.

xli Nadia Oreshkova et.al, "SARS-CoV2 infection in farmed mink, Netherlands, April 2020," *bioRxiv*, May 18, 2020, accessed June 4, 2020, https://doi.org/10.1101/2020.05.18.101493.

xlii International Society for Infectious Diseases, "An update letter from the Minister of Agriculture to the Dutch House of Representatives," Program for Monitoring Emerging Diseases, last modified May 25, 2020, accessed June 4, 2020, https://promedmail.org/promed-post/?id=20200525.7375359.

xliii Sia, S.F., Yan, L., Chin, A.W.H. et.al, "Pathogenesis and transmission of SARS-CoV-2 in golden hamsters," *Nature*, May 14, 2020, accessed June 4, 2020, https://doi.org/10.1038/s41586-020-2342-5.

xliv Camilla Hogdson, "Mystery of prolonged Covid-19 symptoms adds to unknowns," *Financial Times*, May 16, 2020, accessed June 4, 2020, https://www.ft.com/content/91e4482e-d120-49ab-93e3-d314d99b5336.

xlv Roni Caryn Rabin, "What Is 'Covid Toe'? Maybe a Strange Sign of Coronavirus Infection," *New York Times*, May 5, 2020, accessed June 4, 2020, https://www.nytimes.com/2020/05/01/health/coronavirus-covid-toe.html?smid=em-share.

xlvi World Health Organization, "Report of the WHO-China," World Health Organization.

xlvii Ed Yong, "COVID-19 Can Last for Several Months," *The Atlantic*, June 4, 2020, accessed July 14, 2020, https://www.theatlantic.com/health/archive/2020/06/covid-19-coronavirus-longterm-symptoms-months/612679/?utm_source=atl&utm_medium=email&utm_campaign=share.

xlviii Cassandra Willyard, "Coronavirus blood-clot mystery intensifies," *Nature*, May 8, 2020, accessed June 4, 2020, https://www.nature.com/articles/d41586-020-01403-8.

xlix "Blood thinners being used to mitigate risk of clots in COVID-19 patients," CBS News, last modified May 26, 2020, accessed June 4, 2020, https://www.cbsnews.com/news/coronavirus-blood-clots-covid-19-symptom-strokes-young-people/.

l Brian Vastag and Beth Mazur, "Researchers warn covid-19 could cause debilitating long-term illness in some patients," *Washington Post*, May 30, 2020, accessed June 4, 2020, https://www.washingtonpost.com/health/could-covid-19-cause-long-term-chronic-fatigue-and-illness-in-some-patients/2020/05/29/bcd5edb2-a02c-11ea-b5c9-570a91917d8d_story.html.

li Ying Jie Chee, Shereen Jia Huey, and Ester Yeoha, "Diabetic ketoacidosis precipitated by Covid-19 in a patient with newly diagnosed diabetes mellitus," *Diabetes Research and Clinical Practice*, April 24, 2020, accessed July 14, 2020, https://doi.org/10.1016/j.diabres.2020.108166.

lii Smriti Mallapaty, "Mounting clues suggest the coronavirus might trigger diabetes," *Nature*, June 24, 2020, accessed July 14, 2020, https://www.nature.com/articles/d41586-020-01891-8.

liii Ross W Paterson et.al, "The emerging spectrum of COVID-19 neurology: clinical, radiological and laboratory findings," *Brain*, July 8, 2020, accessed July 14, 2020, https://doi.org/10.1093/brain/awaa240.

liv Centers for Disease Control and Prevention, "Groups at Higher Risk for Severe Illness," Centers for Disease Control and Prevention - Coronavirus Disease 2019 (COVID-19), last modified May 14, 2020, accessed June 4, 2020, https://www.cdc.gov/coronavirus/2019-ncov/need-extra-precautions/groups-at-higher-risk.html.

lv World Health Organization, "WHO statement: Tobacco use and COVID-19," World Health Organization, last modified May 11, 2020, accessed June 4, 2020, https://www.who.int/news-room/detail/11-05-2020-who-statement-tobacco-use-and-covid-19.

lvi Centers for Disease Control and Prevention, "People of Any Age with Underlying Medical Conditions," Centers for Disease Control and Prevention - Coronavirus Disease 2019 (COVID-19), last modified June 25, 2020, accessed July 14, 2020, https://www.cdc.gov/coronavirus/2019-ncov/need-extra-precautions/people-with-medical-conditions.html.

lvii Centers for Disease Control and Prevention, "People of Any Age with Underlying Medical Conditions," Centers for Disease Control and Prevention - Coronavirus Disease 2019 (COVID-19), last modified June 25, 2020, accessed July 14, 2020, https://www.cdc.gov/coronavirus/2019-ncov/need-extra-precautions/people-with-medical-conditions.html.

lviii Helen Branswell, "New reports raise possibility pregnant women can pass coronavirus to fetus, but risk is unclear," *STAT News*, March 26, 2020, accessed July 14, 2020, https://www.statnews.com/2020/03/26/new-reports-raise-possibility-pregnant-women-can-pass-coronavirus-to-fetus-but-risk-is-unclear/.

[lix] Kate F. Walker et al., "Maternal transmission of SARS-COV-2 to the neonate, and possible routes for such transmission: A systematic review and critical analysis," *Search Results Web Result with Site Links BJOG: An International Journal of Obstetrics & Gynaecology*, June 12, 2020, accessed July 14, 2020, https://doi.org/10.1111/1471-0528.16362.

[lx] Sascha Ellington et.al, "Characteristics of Women of Reproductive Age with Laboratory-Confirmed SARS-CoV-2 Infection by Pregnancy Status — United States, January 22–June 7, 2020," Morbidity and Mortality Weekly Report (MMWR), last modified June 26, 2020, accessed July 14, 2020, https://www.cdc.gov/mmwr/volumes/69/wr/mm6925a1.htm.

[lxi] Associated Press, "Study suggests fetal coronavirus infection is possible," *Modern Healthcare*, July 10, 2020, accessed July 14, 2020, https://www.modernhealthcare.com/safety-quality/study-suggests-fetal-coronavirus-infection-possible.

[lxii] Huijun Chen et.al, "Clinical characteristics and intrauterine vertical transmission potential of COVID-19 infection in nine pregnant women: a retrospective review of medical records," *The Lancet* 395, no. 10226 (February 12, 2020), accessed July 14, 2020, https://doi.org/10.1016/S0140-6736(20)30360-3.

[lxiii] Kristi Watterberg and COMMITTEE ON FETUS AND NEWBORN, "Providing Care for Infants Born at Home," *Pediatrics* 145, no. 5 (May 2020), accessed June 4, 2020, https://doi.org/10.1542/peds.2020-0626.

[lxiv] March of Dimes, "Coronavirus Disease (COVID-19): What You Need to Know About Its Impact on Moms and Babies," March of Dimes, last modified May 29, 2020, accessed June 4, 2020, https://www.marchofdimes.org/complications/coronavirus-disease-covid-19-what-you-need-to-know.aspx.

lxv Yuanyuan Dong et.al, "Epidemiology of COVID-19 Among Children in China," *Pediatrics* 145, no. 6 (June 2020), accessed July 14, 2020, https://doi.org/10.1542/peds.2020-0702.

lxvi Centers for Disease Control and Prevention, "Evaluation and Management Considerations for Neonates At Risk for COVID-19," Centers for Disease Control and Prevention - Coronavirus Disease 2019 (COVID-19), last modified May 20, 2020, accessed July 14, 2020, https://www.cdc.gov/coronavirus/2019-ncov/hcp/caring-for-newborns.html.

lxvii Aaron E. Carroll, "When Can Grandparents Meet the Newborn?," *New York Times*, June 16, 2020, accessed July 14, 2020, https://www.nytimes.com/2020/06/16/parenting/baby/grandparents-meet-newborn-coronavirus.html.

lxviii David Leffler, "Coronavirus placing high stress on new, expecting moms and raising risks for mental health issues," *Washington Post*, June 21, 2020, accessed July 14, 2020, https://www.washingtonpost.com/health/coronavirus-placing-high-stress-on-new-expecting-moms-and-raising-risks-for-mental-health-issues/2020/06/18/1f5649c6-aa66-11ea-a9d9-a81c1a491c52_story.html.

lxix Centers for Disease Control and Prevention, "For Parents: Multisystem Inflammatory Syndrome in Children (MIS-C) associated with COVID-19," Centers for Disease Control and Prevention - Coronavirus Disease 2019 (COVID-19), https://www.cdc.gov/coronavirus/2019-ncov/daily-life-coping/children/mis-c.html.

lxx Omar Abdel-Mannan et.al, "Neurologic and Radiographic Findings Associated With COVID-19 Infection in Children," *JAMA Neurology*, July 1, 2020, accessed July 14, 2020, https://doi.org/10.1001/jamaneurol.2020.2687.

lxxi Xiaofang Cai et al., "Clinical Characteristics of 5 COVID-19 Cases With Non-respiratory Symptoms as the First Manifestation in Children," *Frontiers in Pediatrics*, May 12, 2020, accessed June 4, 2020, https://doi.org/10.3389/fped.2020.00258.

lxxii Centers for Disease Control and Prevention, "When You Can be Around Others After You Had or Likely Had COVID-19," Centers for Disease Control and Prevention - Coronavirus Disease 2019 (COVID-19), last modified May 26, 2020, accessed July 14, 2020, https://www.cdc.gov/coronavirus/2019-ncov/if-you-are-sick/end-home-isolation.html.

lxxiii Kirkcaldy, King, and Brooks, "COVID-19 and Postinfection".

lxxiv Altmann, Douek, and Boyton, "What policy".

lxxv Quan-Xin Long et.al, "Clinical and immunological assessment of asymptomatic SARS-CoV-2 infections," *Nature Medicine*, June 18, 2020, accessed July 14, 2020, https://doi.org/10.1038/s41591-020-0965-6.

lxxvi Daniel M. Altmann, Daniel C. Douek, and Rosemary J. Boyton, "What policy makers need to know about COVID-19 protective immunity," *The Lancet* 395, no. 10236 (May 16, 2020), accessed June 4, 2020, https://doi.org/10.1016/S0140-6736(20)30985-5.

lxxvii Robert D. Kirkcaldy, Brian A. King, and John T. Brooks, "COVID-19 and Postinfection Immunity: Limited Evidence, Many Remaining Questions," *JAMA*, May 11, 2020, accessed June 4, 2020, https://doi.org/10.1001/jama.2020.7869.

lxxviii Mario Koran, "'It's irresponsible': Washington state warns against 'coronavirus parties,'" *The Guardian*, May 6, 2020, accessed June 4, 2020, https://www.theguardian.com/world/2020/may/06/its-irresponsible-washington-state-sees-sudden-rise-in-covid-parties.

lxxix Jeffrey Seow et.al, "Longitudinal evaluation and decline of antibody responses in SARS-CoV-2 infection," *medRxiv*, July 11, 2020, accessed July 14, 2020, https://doi.org/10.1101/2020.07.09.20148429.

lxxx William A. Haseltine, "Why America Is Losing to COVID-19," *Project Syndicate*, March 31, 2020, accessed June 4, 2020, https://www.project-syndicate.org/commentary/united-states-covid-testing-contact-tracing-by-william-a-haseltine-2020-03.

lxxxi Yasheng Huang, Meicen Sun, and Yuze Sui, "How Digital Contact Tracing Slowed Covid-19 in East Asia," *Harvard Business Review*, April 15, 2020, accessed June 4, 2020, https://hbr.org/2020/04/how-digital-contact-tracing-slowed-covid-19-in-east-asia.

lxxxii Centers for Disease Control and Prevention, "Quarantine and isolation," Centers for Disease Control and Prevention - Quarantine and Isolation, last modified September 29, 2017, accessed July 14, 2020, https://www.cdc.gov/quarantine/index.html.

lxxxiii William A. Haseltine, "How Antibody Tests Can Be Used To Fight COVID-19," *Forbes*, April 6, 2020, accessed June 4, 2020, https://www.forbes.com/sites/williamhaseltine/2020/04/06/how-antibody-tests-can-be-used-to-fight-covid-19/#70c7b57a3904.

lxxxiv Julie Appleby, "What Takes So Long? A Behind-The-Scenes Look At The Steps Involved In COVID-19 Testing," *Kaiser Health News*, May 30, 2020, accessed June 4, 2020, https://khn.org/news/what-takes-so-long-a-behind-the-scenes-look-at-the-steps-involved-in-covid-19-testing/.

lxxxv World Health Organization, "Advice on the use of point-of-care immunodiagnostic tests for COVID-19," World Health Organization, last modified April 8, 2020, accessed June 4, 2020, https://www.who.int/news-room/commentaries/detail/advice-on-the-use-of-point-of-care-immunodiagnostic-tests-for-covid-19.

lxxxvi Stephen M. Hahn and Jeffrey E. Shuren, "Coronavirus (COVID-19) Update: FDA Authorizes First Antigen Test to Help in the Rapid Detection of the Virus that Causes COVID-19 in Patients," U.S. Food & Drug Administration, last modified May 9, 2020, accessed June 4, 2020, https://www.fda.gov/news-events/press-announcements/coronavirus-covid-19-update-fda-authorizes-first-antigen-test-help-rapid-detection-virus-causes.

lxxxvii Neel V. Patel, "Antigen testing could be a faster, cheaper way to diagnose covid-19," *MIT Technology Review*, April 24, 2020, accessed June 4, 2020, https://www.technologyreview.com/2020/04/24/1000486/antigen-testing-could-faster-cheaper-diagnose-covid-19-coronavirus/.

lxxxviii Amir Khan, "Doctor's Note: What are serology tests and do they work?," *Al Jazeera*, May 9, 2020, accessed June 4, 2020, https://www.aljazeera.com/indepth/features/doctor-note-serology-tests-work-200505151942226.html.

lxxxix Alexander Spinelli, "Recovery from Covid-19 is filled with uncertainty. An antibody test offered me a little comfort," *STAT News*, May 21, 2020, accessed June 4, 2020, https://www.statnews.com/2020/05/21/recovery-from-covid-19-antibodies-uncertainty/.

xc Nicoletta Lanese, "First at-home saliva test for COVID-19 earns FDA approval," Live Science, last modified May 2020, accessed June 4, 2020, https://www.livescience.com/at-home-saliva-test-for-covid19.html.

xci U.S. Food & Drug Administration, "Coronavirus (COVID-19) Update: FDA Issues Warning Letters to Companies Inappropriately Marketing Antibody Tests, Potentially Placing Public Health at Risk," FDA Newsroom, last modified June 17, 2020, accessed July 14, 2020, https://www.fda.gov/news-events/press-announcements/coronavirus-covid-19-update-fda-issues-warning-letters-companies-inappropriately-marketing-antibody.

[xcii] Drew Harwell, "Thermal scanners are the latest technology being deployed to detect the coronavirus. But they don't really work.," *Washington Post*, May 11, 2020, accessed June 4, 2020, https://www.washingtonpost.com/technology/2020/05/11/thermal-scanners-are-latest-technology-being-deployed-detect-coronavirus-they-dont-really-work/.

[xciii] Katelyn Gostic et al., "Estimated effectiveness of symptom and risk screening to prevent the spread of COVID-19," *eLife Sciences*, February 24, 2020, accessed June 4, 2020, https://doi.org/10.7554/eLife.55570.

[xciv] Centers for Disease Control and Prevention, "Community Transmission of SARS-CoV-2 at Two Family Gatherings — Chicago, Illinois, February–March 2020," Morbidity and Mortality Weekly Report (MMWR), last modified April 17, 2020, accessed June 4, 2020, https://www.cdc.gov/mmwr/volumes/69/wr/mm6915e1.htm?s_cid=mm6915e1_w.

[xcv] Eric Holdeman, "COVID-19: Transmission Scenarios Explained," *Government Technology*, May 11, 2020, accessed June 4, 2020, https://www.govtech.com/em/emergency-blogs/disaster-zone/covid-19-transmission-scenarios-explained.html.

[xcvi] Bruce Y. Lee, "Where Coronavirus Is More Likely To Be Airborne, 5 Places To Avoid," *Forbes*, May 30, 2020, accessed June 4, 2020, https://www.forbes.com/sites/brucelee/2020/05/30/where-coronavirus-is-more-likely-to-be-airborne-5-places-to-avoid/#44f194bb39ab.

[xcvii] California State Government, "Stay home Q&A," Covid19.CA.gov, last modified June 4, 2020, accessed June 4, 2020, https://covid19.ca.gov/stay-

home-except-for-essential-needs/?campaign_id=49&emc=edit_ca_20200501&instance_id=18134&nl=california-today®i_id=78159988&segment_id=26374&te=1&user_id=930b2d6d815949d1bd3f3835944a4f18#outdoor.

[xcviii] Centers for Disease Control and Prevention, "Visiting Parks and Recreational Facilities," Centers for Disease Control and Prevention - Coronavirus Disease 2019 (COVID-19), last modified May 19, 2020, accessed June 4, 2020, https://www.cdc.gov/coronavirus/2019-ncov/daily-life-coping/visitors.html.

[xcix] California State Government, "Stay home," Covid19.CA.gov.

[c] Beth Teitell, "We can take road trips now. But where are we supposed to go to the bathroom?," *Boston Globe*, June 8, 2020, accessed July 14, 2020, https://www.bostonglobe.com/2020/06/08/nation/we-can-take-road-trips-now-where-are-we-supposed-go-bathroom/.

[ci] James Paton, Jason Gale, and John Lauerman, "The Race to Develop a Coronavirus Vaccine: What you need to know," *Bloomberg*, May 8, 2020, accessed May 29, 2020, https://www.bloomberg.com/news/storythreads/2020-05-08/the-race-to-develop-a-coronavirus-vaccine.

[cii] "Does the flu vaccine work as well in elderly people?," *Harvard Health Publishing*, December 2019, accessed May 29, 2020, https://www.health.harvard.edu/diseases-and-conditions/does-the-flu-vaccine-work-as-well-in-elderly-people.

[ciii] Centers for Disease Control and Prevention, "Vaccination of Tier 1 at All Pandemic Severities," Centers for Disease Control and Prevention - Influenza (Flu), last modified October 24, 2018, accessed May 29, 2020,

https://www.cdc.gov/flu/pandemic-resources/national-strategy/planning-guidance/pandemic-severities-tier-1.html.

[civ] James Gallagher, "Coronavirus cure: When will we have a drug to treat it?," *BBC News*, May 27, 2020, accessed June 4, 2020, https://www.bbc.com/news/health-52354520.

[cv] Andrés Pizzorno et al., "Drug Repurposing Approaches for the Treatment of Influenza Viral Infection: Reviving Old Drugs to Fight Against a Long-Lived Enemy," *Frontiers in Immunology* 10, no. 531 (March 19, 2020), accessed May 29, 2020, https://doi.org/10.3389/fimmu.2019.00531.

[cvi] Duan, Kai et.al, "The feasibility".

[cvii] U.S. Food & Drug Administration, "FDA COMBATING COVID-19 WITH THERAPEUTICS," U.S. Food & Drug Administration, last modified May 11, 2020, accessed June 4, 2020, https://www.fda.gov/media/136832/download.

[cviii] Kay Lazar and Andrew Ryan, "No, warm weather will not kill the coronavirus," *Boston Globe*, April 24, 2020, accessed June 4, 2020, https://www.bostonglobe.com/2020/04/24/nation/no-warm-weather-will-not-kill-coronavirus/.

[cix] The Scripps Research Institute, "Mutated coronavirus shows significant boost in infectivity," Scripps Research, last modified June 12, 2020, accessed July 14, 2020, https://www.scripps.edu/news-and-events/press-room/2020/20200612-choe-farzan-coronavirus-spike-mutation.html.

[cx] National Institutes of Health, "COVID-19, MERS & SARS," National Institute of Allergy and Infectious Diseases - Coronavirus, last modified April 6, 2020, accessed July 14, 2020, https://www.niaid.nih.gov/diseases-conditions/covid-19.

[cxi] Zhou, Hong et.al, "A Novel Bat Coronavirus Closely Related to SARS-CoV-2 Contains Natural Insertions at the S1/S2 Cleavage Site of the Spike Protein," *Current Biology*, May 10, 2020, accessed June 4, 2020, https://doi.org/10.1016/j.cub.2020.05.023.

[cxii] National Institutes of Health, "NIAID Emerging Infectious Diseases/ Pathogens," National Institute of Allergy and Infectious Disease - Biodefense, last modified July 26, 2018, accessed June 4, 2020, https://www.niaid.nih.gov/research/emerging-infectious-diseases-pathogens.

[cxiii] University of Oxford, "Co-SPACE study - COVID-19: Supporting Parents, Adolescents, and Children during Epidemics," Department of Experimental Psychology at University of Oxford, accessed June 4, 2020, https://oxfordxpsy.az1.qualtrics.com/jfe/form/SV_3VO130LTKOcloMd.

[cxiv] Oliver Franklin-Wallis, "How School Shutdowns Have Long-Term Effects on Children," *WIRED UK*, May 18, 2020, accessed June 4, 2020, https://www.wired.com/story/how-school-shutdowns-have-longterm-effects-on-children/?utm_source=onsite-share&utm_medium=email&utm_campaign=onsite-share&utm_brand=wired.

[cxv] Carl Cullinane and Rebecca Montacute, "COVID-19 and Social Mobility Impact Brief #1: School Shutdown," The Sutton Trust, last modified April 2020, accessed June 4, 2020, https://www.suttontrust.com/wp-content/uploads/2020/04/COVID-19-Impact-Brief-School-Shutdown.pdf.

[cxvi] "Coronavirus: Lessons From Asia," *Al Jazeera*, May 3, 2020, accessed June 4, 2020, https://www.aljazeera.com/programmes/specialseries/2020/05/coronavirus-lessons-asia-200501110507558.html.

cxvii Chelsea Janes, "In some nations, government isolation centers helped reduce coronavirus infections. The U.S. has resisted the strategy.," *Washington Post*, May 20, 2020, accessed June 4, 2020, https://www.washingtonpost.com/health/in-some-nations-government-isolation-centers-helped-reduce-covid-19-infections-the-us-has-resisted-the-strategy/2020/05/19/533850d6-9616-11ea-9f5e-56d8239bf9ad_story.html.

cxviii Heather Landi, "Half of physicians now using telehealth as COVID-19 changes practice operations," *Fierce Healthcare*, April 23, 2020, accessed June 4, 2020, https://www.fiercehealthcare.com/practices/half-physicians-now-using-telehealth-as-covid-changes-practice-operations.

cxix Ateev Mehrotra et al., "The Impact of the COVID-19 Pandemic on Outpatient Visits: A Rebound Emerges," The Commonwealth Fund, last modified May 19, 2020, accessed June 4, 2020, https://www.commonwealthfund.org/publications/2020/apr/impact-covid-19-outpatient-visits.

cxx Blue Cross Blue Shield of Massachusetts, "Blue Cross Blue Shield of Massachusetts Processes 1 Million Telehealth Claims in 9 Weeks," Blue Cross Blue Shield of Massachusetts, last modified May 21, 2020, accessed June 4, 2020, http://newsroom.bluecrossma.com/2020-05-21-Blue-Cross-Blue-Shield-of-Massachusetts-Processes-1-Million-Telehealth-Claims-in-9-Weeks?utm_source=STAT+Newsletters&utm_campaign=ff37996f74-MR_COPY_01&utm_medium=email&utm_term=0_8cab1d7961-ff37996f74-151227717.

cxxi Bertha Coombs, "Telehealth visits are booming as doctors and patients embrace distancing amid the coronavirus crisis," CNBC, last modified April 4, 2020, accessed June 4, 2020,

https://www.cnbc.com/2020/04/03/telehealth-visits-could-top-1-billion-in-2020-amid-the-coronavirus-crisis.html.

cxxii Francesco Cirillo, "The Pomodoro Technique®," The Pomodoro Technique®, last modified 2020, accessed June 4, 2020, https://francescocirillo.com/pages/pomodoro-technique.

cxxiii Hiroshi Nishiura et al., "Closed environments facilitate secondary transmission of coronavirus disease 2019 (COVID-19)," *medRxiv*, April 16, 2020, accessed July 14, 2020, https://doi.org/10.1101/2020.02.28.20029272.

cxxiv Hua Qian et al., "Indoor transmission of SARS-CoV-2," *medRxiv*, April 7, 2020, accessed July 14, 2020, https://doi.org/10.1101/2020.04.04.20053058.

cxxv U.S. Centers for Disease Control and Prevention, "Considerations for Public Pools, Hot Tubs, and Water Playgrounds During COVID-19," Centers for Disease Control and Prevention - Coronavirus Disease 2019 (COVID-19), last modified May 27, 2020, accessed July 14, 2020, https://www.cdc.gov/coronavirus/2019-ncov/community/parks-rec/aquatic-venues.html.

cxxvi U.S. Centers for Disease Control and Prevention, "Personal and Social Activities," Centers for Disease Control and Prevention - Coronavirus Disease 2019 (COVID-19), last modified June 15, 2020, accessed July 14, 2020, https://www.cdc.gov/coronavirus/2019-ncov/daily-life-coping/personal-social-activities.html.

cxxvii U.S. Centers for Disease Control and Prevention, "Personal and Social Activities," Centers for Disease Control and Prevention - Coronavirus Disease 2019 (COVID-19), last modified June 15, 2020, accessed July 14, 2020, https://www.cdc.gov/coronavirus/2019-ncov/daily-life-coping/personal-social-activities.html.

cxxviii U.S. Centers for Disease Control and Prevention, "Personal and Social Activities," Centers for Disease Control and Prevention - Coronavirus Disease 2019 (COVID-19), last modified June 15, 2020, accessed July 14, 2020, https://www.cdc.gov/coronavirus/2019-ncov/daily-life-coping/personal-social-activities.html.

cxxix Tara Parker-Pope, "How Safe Are Outdoor Gatherings?," *New York Times*, July 3, 2020, accessed July 14, 2020, https://www.nytimes.com/2020/07/03/well/live/coronavirus-spread-outdoors-party.html?smid=em-share.

cxxx U.S. Centers for Disease Control and Prevention, "Personal and Social Activities," Centers for Disease Control and Prevention - Coronavirus Disease 2019 (COVID-19), last modified June 15, 2020, accessed July 14, 2020, https://www.cdc.gov/coronavirus/2019-ncov/daily-life-coping/personal-social-activities.html.

cxxxi Hilary Potkewitz, "How to Exercise Safely Outdoors in the Heat," *Wall Street Journal*, July 12, 2020, accessed July 14, 2020, https://www.wsj.com/articles/how-to-exercise-safely-outdoors-in-the-heat-11594551600?st=juvahmsij2hrnci&reflink=article_email_share.

cxxxii U.S. Centers for Disease Control and Prevention, "Visiting Parks and Recreational Facilities," Centers for Disease Control and Prevention - Coronavirus Disease 2019 (COVID-19), last modified June 9, 2020, accessed July 14, 2020, https://www.cdc.gov/coronavirus/2019-ncov/daily-life-coping/visitors.html.

cxxxiii Christina Caron, "As Playgrounds Start to Reopen, Here's How to Keep Kids Safe," *New York Times*, June 11, 2020, accessed July 14, 2020, https://www.nytimes.com/2020/06/11/parenting/playgrounds-reopen-safety-coronavirus.html?smid=em-share.

cxxxiv Harvard Medical School, "Coronavirus outbreak and kids," Harvard Health Publishing, last modified July 2, 2020, accessed July 14, 2020, https://www.health.harvard.edu/diseases-and-conditions/coronavirus-outbreak-and-kids.

cxxxv Fei Xiao et al., "Infectious SARS-CoV-2 in Feces of Patient with Severe COVID-19," *Emerging Infectious Diseases* 26, no. 8 (August 2020), accessed July 14, 2020, https://doi.org/10.3201/eid2608.200681.

cxxxvi U.S. Centers for Disease Control and Prevention, "Considerations for Public Pools, Hot Tubs, and Water Playgrounds During COVID-19," Centers for Disease Control and Prevention - Coronavirus Disease 2019 (COVID-19), last modified May 27, 2020, accessed July 14, 2020, https://www.cdc.gov/coronavirus/2019-ncov/community/parks-rec/aquatic-venues.html.

cxxxvii U.S. Centers for Disease Control and Prevention, "Considerations for Public Beaches," Centers for Disease Control and Prevention - Coronavirus Disease 2019 (COVID-19), last modified June 16, 2020, accessed July 14, 2020, https://www.cdc.gov/coronavirus/2019-ncov/community/parks-rec/public-beaches.html.

cxxxviii U.S. Centers for Disease Control and Prevention, "Suggestions for Youth and Summer Camps," Centers for Disease Control and Prevention - Coronavirus Disease 2019 (COVID-19), last modified June 25, 2020, accessed July 14, 2020, https://www.cdc.gov/coronavirus/2019-ncov/community/schools-childcare/summer-camps.html.

cxxxix Beth Teitell, "We can take road trips now. But where are we supposed to go to the bathroom?," *Boston Globe*, June 8, 2020, accessed July 14, 2020, https://www.bostonglobe.com/2020/06/08/nation/we-can-take-road-trips-now-where-are-we-supposed-go-bathroom/.

cxl Christopher Elliott, "Everything Americans need to know about the E.U. travel ban," *Washington Post*, July 8, 2020, accessed July 14, 2020, https://www.washingtonpost.com/lifestyle/travel/everything-americans-need-to-know-about-the-eu-travel-ban/2020/07/08/8fea554e-bc89-11ea-80b9-40ece9a701dc_story.html.

cxli European Commission, "Travel to and from the EU during the pandemic," European Commission website, last modified June 2020, accessed July 14, 2020, https://ec.europa.eu/info/live-work-travel-eu/health/coronavirus-response/travel-and-transportation-during-coronavirus-pandemic/travel-and-eu-during-pandemic_en#exemption-details.

CPSIA information can be obtained
at www.ICGtesting.com
Printed in the USA
LVHW070032110820
662834LV00023B/2638